Mohamed Islam Kediha

Cognition and multiple sclerosis: diagnosis and management

Mohamed Islam Kediha

Cognition and multiple sclerosis: diagnosis and management

ScienciaScripts

Imprint

Any brand names and product names mentioned in this book are subject to trademark, brand or patent protection and are trademarks or registered trademarks of their respective holders. The use of brand names, product names, common names, trade names, product descriptions etc. even without a particular marking in this work is in no way to be construed to mean that such names may be regarded as unrestricted in respect of trademark and brand protection legislation and could thus be used by anyone.

Cover image: www.ingimage.com

This book is a translation from the original published under ISBN 978-620-6-72100-0.

Publisher:
Sciencia Scripts
is a trademark of
Dodo Books Indian Ocean Ltd. and OmniScriptum S.R.L publishing group

120 High Road, East Finchley, London, N2 9ED, United Kingdom
Str. Armeneasca 28/1, office 1, Chisinau MD-2012, Republic of Moldova, Europe
Printed at: see last page
ISBN: 978-620-8-08383-0

FOREWORD

Since the first descriptions of multiple sclerosis in the second half of the nineteenth century, the diagnostic criteria, the means of diagnosis and the treatment have all changed. and therapeutic potential have never ceased to evolve.

Cognitive disorders in this increasingly common condition, which for a long time were wrongly regarded as secondary signs and even sometimes described as invisible signs, have aroused a great deal of interest and have been the subject of numerous studies in recent years.

In the current evolution of neurological practice and the management of patients with multiple sclerosis, numerous neuropsychological tests have been validated and submitted to patients, giving neurologists a better understanding of their cognitive disorders.

This book provides clear, in-depth illustrations of the main forms of cognitive impairment in multiple sclerosis.

From a diagnostic perspective, the author uses a number of case studies to present the main features of these disorders, particularly in Algerian patients, as well as some unusual aspects of this type of brain damage.

Neurologists should find it of definite interest in their daily practice.

Professor Lamia Ali Pacha

CONTENTS

INTRODUCTION

Multiple sclerosis (MS) is the most common demyelinating disease of the central nervous system (CNS), and the main cause of neurological disability in young adults. It is considered to be one of the most common acquired neurological diseases of young people, with life-long projects. It develops in a chronic mode, and the clinical picture may include various neurological symptoms and signs, which reflect the distribution of the various lesions of demyelination observed. Clinicians have always focused on the physical aspects of the disease. Nevertheless, many non-motor signs such as genito- sphincter disorders, fatigue, anxiety, depressive syndrome, psychiatric disorders and cognitive disorders are very common. of the disease. [1]. These symptoms are rarely reported by patients, as they are often hidden or even drowned out by other physical symptoms. According to two French studies [2,3], 40-65% of patients suffer from cognitive disorders; these are the 1[ers] studies that have raised the possibility that these disorders are ultimately frequent clinical manifestations of MS. This will result in a source of isolation, leading to a kind of double punishment, both motor and cognitive, described as a "mental illness". "mental wheelchair". These disorders affect patients' daily lives, with a negative impact on their quality of life (QoL) [4].

Since the early 1980s, the use of neuropsychological tests in MS has become routine, as has the advent of magnetic resonance imaging (MRI). These two factors have greatly improved our understanding of cognitive impairment in MS [4].In view of the recent renewed interest in these signs and the increasingly frequent complaints from patients to specialist clinics, clinicians are in a difficult position to respond to the needs of their patients. the need to attach greater importance to them, especially as they are associated with social and professional repercussions such as loss of employment [5]. The Screening for these disorders is therefore important, and neurologists must invest in their assessment in order to offer appropriate treatment. Cognitive impairment (CIA) can be seen at all stages of MS, particularly in the most severe cases.such as clinically isolated syndromes (CIS) and radiologically isolated syndromes (RIS) [6]. This highlights the importance of early detection of these disorders with adapted psycho-cognitive tools [7].

Information processing speed (IPT) and working memory are the areas where the brain is most active. cognitive problems most frequently affected [8]. Various assessment tools can be used to evaluate cognitive impairment in people with MS. A short, reproducible battery specific to MS was proposed in 1989 and

validated in French in 2004 under the name Batterie Courte d'évaluation des fonctions cognitives (BCCog-SEP) [9,10]. This was the first neuropsychological test battery validated in MS.
different batteries subsequently validated in their exploration. It should be noted that many arguments underline the importance of this neuropsychological assessment. The disorders
may be associated with depression, unemployment, reduced social interaction, inability to drive and deterioration in QoL. [11, 12].

Early detection of cognitive disorders and monitoring of their progress enable neuropsychological intervention programmes and psychological therapies to be proposed. [13, 14].
In addition, the way the disease is portrayed and its unpredictable course can have a significant impact on the quality of life of patients.

impact on future projection and weaken self-esteem and self-confidence, leading to anxiety and depression. Anxiety and depression are symptoms of
common in MS that need to be taken into account. In addition, the presence of cognitive problems can be considered as a long-term prognostic factor, having an implication in
the choice of disease-modifying treatments and enabling a reliable assessment of the EDSS (Expanded Disability Status Scale) functional score in the monitoring of disability. [15, 16].

Among the cognitive dysfunctions observed in people with MS, it has been reported that they affect not only perceptual-motor functions, but also language, memory and memory. working memory, sustained attention, information processing speed and executive functions, but also social cognition (SC) [17].

Social cognition encompasses the mental operations that underlie interactions between people. including the ability to perceive, interpret and generate responses to social events. intentions, dispositions and behaviours of others. This definition makes it possible to from broader cognitive functions such as memory, attention and the functions of the brain. executive functions, which are generally affected by cognitive disorders [18]. A chapter will be devoted to this in this book.

Very few studies have been carried out using unselected samples of patients recruited consecutively from the general population, to assess the effectiveness of the treatment. actual frequency of cognitive impairment. The study by Rao et al [2] used a very large battery comprising 31 scores in 100 MS patients recruited from the general population, compared with 100 matched healthy controls. Forty-three percent of MS patients had abnormal results on at least 4 scores, mainly affecting short-term memory, sustained attention, verbal fluency and reasoning. On the basis of these data, Rao et al [2] proposed a brief screening battery (20 to 30 minutes to complete) comprising 4 tests. Another study, by McIntosh Michaelis et al [19], found that 46% of patients in a sample of 147 had cognitive problems.These cognitive problems are frequent or frequently reported symptoms. by MS patients, with a prevalence of around 50 to 60%. These disorders have an impact on the general quality of social life [20].

Cognitive deficits may appear in the early stages of the disease, even in the absence of other neurological manifestations. This was demonstrated in a study Kediha et al [21]. In this study, the cognitive performance of a group of patients presenting with a 1[er] demyelinating event or CIS was evaluated, and the main domains that would be most affected at an early stage in this condition were identified. identified. Patient data was compared with that of a control group with the same epidemiological characteristics as part of a case-control study. The The overall results showed that cognitive impairment was frequent in the CIS group in this series, mainly affecting the speed of VTI information processing (84.6%), followed by visuospatial memory (69.2%), attentional and working memory (53.8%), then language (38.4%) and finally executive functions (30.7%). See figure 1.

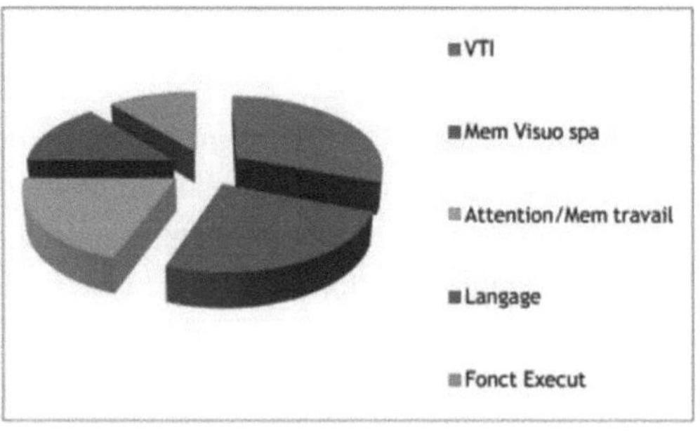

VTI: vitesse de traitement de l'information. Mem: mémoire. Visuo spa: visuo spatiale. Fonct Execut: fonction exécutive.

Figure 1: Major cognitive functions impaired in patients with clinically isolated syndrome (Kediha et al. 2020)[21].

An accurate description and diagnosis of CTs in the early stages of MS is of great importance, as it may determine the effectiveness of the treatment. potential preventive measures, but may also be a predictor of future disease progression [26], but also of poor clinical outcome, and by They should therefore be considered as markers of aggressive forms of this pathology [22].

The cognitive areas most frequently affected are :
- The speed of information processing
- Attention disorders
- Working memory,
- Visual-spatial memory
- Executive functions [23, 24].
There is a predominance of dysexecutive disorders in progressive forms, and an amnestic profile in remittent forms [25].
Furthermore, CT may precede the onset of other MS symptoms by more than a year [26].
Early management of these patients could help improve their quality of life, and even reduce the unemployment rate, which is frequently observed in this group of patients [27, 28].

A Dutch cohort of 234 patients versus 60 control subjects, with a follow-up of 05 years, showed that 28% of these patients developed a cognitive deficit. This deficit was clearly predominant in progressive forms [31].

With regard to the cognitive domains affected during the initial phases of the disease, it is worth noting the following

It would appear that ITV and executive functions are affected first, followed by memory disorders and then attention disorders [21, 29]. Cortical domains (praxias and gnosias) are generally spared, even in the advanced stages of disease [30, 31].

Executive dysfunction is linked to an inability to solve problems and poor task planning. Frequently, the patient has difficulty initiating an action and achieving a goal, or managing transitions to complete the task. The
prolonged concentration is reduced and multitasking is generally impaired. The

Visual and spatial processing is affected, with problems with orientation and navigation. The ability to perceive new information is reduced, as is the ability to learn, understand and use information.
so it is often necessary to hear repeated information. In addition, word fluency is affected and speech is incoherent. [32]

However, fatigue and depression must be taken into account during assessment, as they represent the most common comorbidities in MS and are often confounding factors with the negative impact on cognition. Fatigue is often confused with cognitive impairment. It is subjectively described as a general tiredness and lack of energy. of energy, implying a reduction in the ability to carry out a long-term task. Depression affects almost half of MS patients, and clinically depressed patients often have working memory problems or have difficulty planning and carrying out tasks. [33 ; 26].

Although impairment of cognitive function occurs in a number of different diseasesneurological disorders, the clinical syndromes, the degree of dysfunction and the resulting disability depend on the involvement of different brain structures (cortical or subcortical), the extent of neuronal lesions or the number of areas affected, as well as the patient's previous cognitive reserve and performance. In the case of MS, As a heterogeneous disease, all the above characteristics make it even more difficult to study cognition as a single manifestation of the disease. Despite advances in knowledge about the neural basis of cognitive function in MS, major uncertainties remain about what is termed 'normal cognition' and, consequently, about the assessment of cognitive dysfunction, generally defined as performance below a chosen threshold in a number of cognitive domains, assessed in a specific neuropsychological test (e.g. 1.5 to 2 deviations-types below the normal Z-score for one or more cognitive domains). In these batteries, scores are generally expressed as "intact/preserved" or "impaired" [29], and prevalent studies generally differ in their definitions of impairment cognitive [34, 35]. MS is generally diagnosed during the most productive period of a patient's life, and years of employment and cognitive impairment imply a severe impact on the patient's behaviour, social functioning, coping strategies and profound functional limitations affecting activities of daily living and employment. A vast cross-sectional study carried out in nine European countries showed that only 35.8% of multiple sclerosis patients were employed. Poor mood and cognitive disorders affecting areas such as memory, attention and slowing of speed of information processing were reported as frequent determinants of employment-related difficulties, but only working memory disorders were responsible for higher unemployment rates [36]. Employment offers a better quality of life, independence, social participation, personal and professional reaffirmation, a sense of belonging and a sense of belonging. As a result, preserving cognition should be a priority at a time when highly active treatments are reducing relapses and new lesions, and when new horizons are opening up for preventing the accumulation of Alzheimer's disease.physical disability thanks to new disease-modifying treatments. Lastly, cognitive disorders not only affect patients, but also their relationships with their families, and are often the source of a heavier burden for carers [37].Mickens et al. studied the mediating effect on the relationships between MS impairments (neurological, cognitive, behavioural, emotional and functional), needs unmet family needs (household, financial, social, support and health information) and the carer's mental health (life satisfaction, anxiety, burden and depression). They suggested that intervention research on patient carers could consider focus on the mental health problems of carers by meeting their needs and by teaching carers to manage the impairments of the person with MS [38].

CTs in MS appear to be becoming a frequent clinical manifestation, but their pathophysiology remains incompletely understood. It would appear that lesions of the white matter and grey matter, as well as the synaptic dysfunction play a major role. As a result, the measurement of certain biomarkers in cerebrospinal fluid (CSF), and the study of their association with CT, can provide interesting in vivo evidence that may explain the mechanisms that lead to the development of these disorders.that underlie CT [39]. Therefore, the identification of a biomarker with good diagnostic and prognostic power would be of great importance for the monitoring and prevention of cognitive impairment in MS patients. Some studies have proposed measuring levels of amyloid B protein (AB 42) in CSF (associated with cognitive decline in Alzheimer's disease), combined with synaptic plasticity in the brain, which is a measure of cognitive reserve in humans [40].Various CSF biomarkers are currently being studied and validated. Nevertheless, some of them appear to be closely correlated with CT in MS (see figure 2) [39]. Biomarkers of axonal damage : Although CT in MS is not exclusively related to subcortical lesions, the involvement of white matter remains an important and predominant factor [41]. The most studied biomarker reflecting axonal lesions in various diseases neurotransmitters are light chain neurofilaments (LCNFs) [42]. Changes in NFCL levels are directly related to the ongoing inflammatory axonal damage observed in MS. For these properties, the study of NFCL in the CSF can provide informationIt is interesting to note the contribution of axonal damage to the cognitive deficits associated with the disease. Their rate is significantly higher in people with TC [43].

Biomarkers related to amyloid metabolism :

Cerebral amyloid lesions are a well-known histopathological feature of AD, and are also found in other neurodegenerative diseases [44]. Low levels of AB42 proteins are found in the CSF of MS patients with CTs, and are correlated with a risk of developing them during the course of the disease [45].

Biomarkers associated with intrathecal Ig synthesis :

Oligoclonal bands (OCBs) are currently the only clinically defined biomarker for MS. They are, however, not very specific, as they can be found in a very small number of MS patients. variety of neuroinflammatory diseases [46]. These

BOCs could reflect the severity of the disease and be correlated with poorer cognitive performance. It has recently been shown that MS patients with a positive BOC more frequently present a cognitive deficit compared with the general population [47].

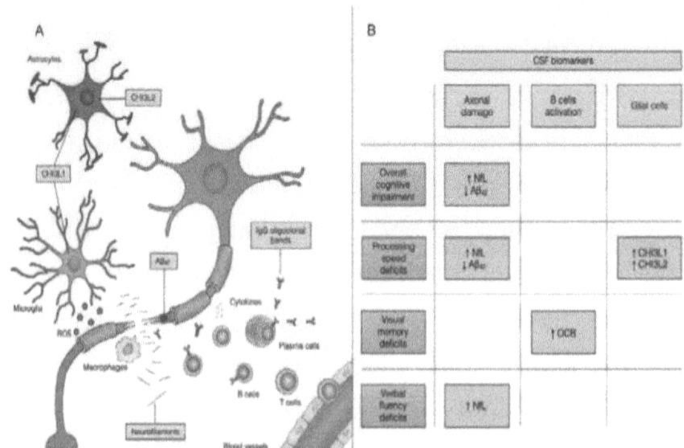

Figure 2: CSF biomarkers in multiple sclerosis: physio-pathological explanations and association with cognitive disorders. [39]

In addition, other factors may be taken into account in the assumptions pathophysiology of cognitive impairment in MS. The newly identified role of the choroid plexuses (CPs) in the pathophysiology of MS is increasingly recognised. Chronic inflammation, which is accompanied by a higher number and volume of Paramagnetic Rim Lesions (PRL) and PC hypertrophy may contribute to cognitive impairment in MS, in addition to grey matter atrophy. The contribution of PC hypertrophy in the explanation of fatigue confirms the importance of immune-related processes in determining this manifestation, independently of the severity of the disease. PRL and PC hypertrophy may contribute to the pathophysiology of cognitive impairment and fatigue in MS. They may represent targets clinically relevant therapies to limit the impact of these clinical manifestations in MS. [48].

Recent MRI studies have demonstrated that complex mechanisms can partly explain cognitive dysfunction in MS [49, 50, 51]. These include a "disconnection syndrome" caused by the accumulation of focal lesions and microstructural tissue abnormalities in cognition-related white matter (WM) pathways, the development of focal and diffuse lesions in strategic grey matter (GM) regions, and the presence of functional abnormalities in the brain network reflecting a progressive failure of the brain's adaptive capacity [52].

Furthermore, recent pathological and MRI studies have confirmed the role of chronic inflammation as one of the most important factors in the more severe progression of disability in MS [53]. In this context, chronic active lesions and enlargement of the choroid plexus have been suggested as two clinically relevant indicators of chronic inflammation that can be explored in vivo using MRI. Chronic active lesions are pathologically characterised by a peripheral 'edge' of activated iron-loaded microglia/macrophages, associated with ongoing demyelination and axonal loss around an inactive nucleus without damage to the blood-brain barrier [54] These lesions have a hypointense paramagnetic rim (i.e. lesions with a paramagnetic rim), which corresponds to the iron-loaded peripheral microglia. In MS, PRLs have been associated with more severe clinical disability, progressive disease progression and cerebral atrophy. PCs play a key role in immunological regulation within the CNS as they act as an interface between the peripheral immune system and the CNS [55]. Significant enlargement of PCs occurs in the early stages of MS and is associated with a higher relapse rate, T2-hyperintense brain lesion volume and inflammatory activity, as well as a more severe progression of disability. [56]. Higher PRL load and PC hypertrophy, reflecting a chronic pro-inflammatory environment, are likely to contribute both to the deterioration of cognitive performance and fatigue, possibly by promoting progressive demyelination, neuro-axonal damage and synaptic loss [57]. However, to date, the relationship between chronic inflammation and cognitive impairment has only been partially explored [58].

MS patients with at least 1 or 4 PRLs [59] showed poorer cognitive performance and reached cognitive impairment at a younger age. We have also found that a significantly higher volume of PCs was associated with poorer cognitive performance.The results of a recent study suggest that a higher load of PRL can characterise MS patients with poorer cognitive performance, confirming the key role of chronic inflammation in the CNS as a driver of more severe disease progression [48]. PC enlargement may therefore be at the origin of structural and functional abnormalities of this structure which reflect a state of chronic inflammation, with abnormal migration, localisation and activation of immune cells within the CNS. These processes can lead to a chronic inflammatory state in the CNS, with higher levels of pro-inflammatory cytokines and chemokines. and lower levels of anti-inflammatory cytokines, such as interleukin 10. The involvement of the choroid plexuses (CPs) in the pathophysiology of MS is increasingly recognised [60]. However, their involvement in the genesis of cognitive disorders has recently been suggested [48].

PCs play a key role in immunological regulation within the CNS as they act as an interface between the peripheral immune system and the CNS [55]. A significant enlargement of the PCs occurs in the early stages of MS and is associated with a higher relapse rate and a higher rate of white matter hypersignals in the brain, as well as an increase in their volume and activity inflammation. All these factors are associated with disability that progresses more severely [56]. It was also found that an increase in the volume of PCs was associated with a deterioration in cognitive performance [61]. Furthermore, MS patients with or without cognitive impairment showed a significant increase in CP volume compared with healthy subjects. It is interesting to note that in the direct comparison MS patients with cognitive impairment showed significantly higher PC volume than cognitively preserved patients. The PC represents a gateway for the entry of lymphocytes from the peripheral blood into the CNS, and is involved in the antigen presentation [62]. The structure and function of capillaries and ependymal cells, including increased permeability of capillaries, thickening of the basement membrane and loss of cilia in ependymal cells, have also been reported. reported [63]. These pathological processes may not only promote demyelination and neuro-axonal loss, but also alter synaptic function, which plays an important role not only in the progression of the disease, but also in cognitive impairment. These MRI biomarkers may represent new therapeutic targets and could be used in the development of new drugs. clinically relevant for future treatments aimed at reducing the adverse effects of MS not only on clinical disability, but also on cognitive impairment and fatigue.

CLINICAL ASPECTS

Faced with a patient and/or his family consulting for possible cognitive impairment, the clinician must take into account psychiatric comorbidities, the side effects of certain medications and certain MS symptoms that could adversely affect cognitive performance, which are the basic principles for assessing and managing cognitive impairment in MS patients. In two large fundamental studies, patients were classified if their performance was impaired in four of the 31 tests used or in two of the 11 tests in a battery of multi-domain neuropsychological tests [63].

Like all the organic symptoms of MS, cognitive impairment is characterised by great variability between patients. Nevertheless, 03 main complaints are found: ITV, learning and memory. Impairment of executive and visuospatial functions is also observed. Furthermore, basic language, semantic memory and attention skills rarely seem to be affected.impaired (10% of MS patients) [63]; but semantic fluency seems to be predominant in the over-50s. Cognitive disorders in MS are essentially based on impairment of the basic neuropsychological foundation of attention. Attention is considered to be a basic function involved in any cognitive performance or behavioural task. It is at the forefront of the cognitive consequences of brain damage. Attention enables selection in perception and action and facilitates the processing of information, hence the very close link between loss of attentional capacity and slowing of VTI [64].
Cognitive complaints affect all progressive forms of MS. This includes CIS, but also radiologically isolated syndromes (RIS). The slowing of ITV is the cognitive hallmark of MS, and this will have a direct impact on certain downstream domains [65].
From an evolutionary point of view, the progression and severity of CDs are highly variable. Some complaints worsen very quickly, others more slowly. The impact on certain activities of life Daily activities will also vary, including work, driving and managing personal finances [66].

These cognitive clinical aspects in MS can be approached from an analytical point of view, with attention being the main area affected. An examination of more than 1100 patients by Sullivan et al [67]. It was deduced that 38% of patients had at least one cognitive impairment and 22% had a predominant impairment of attention. Other studies have also looked at attention disorders in early forms of MS (CIS stage). These include the Algerian study by Kediha et al [21], which had found attentional disorders in a case-control study; but also the

Callanan et al study [68], which showed that CIS patients had an impairment of significantly greater for visual and auditory attention. Furthermore, it is clear that patients have difficulty using significant attentional resources during certain executive tasks, as illustrated by the study by Graffman et al [69] who compared 41 MS patients with 45 control subjects for certain memory tasks. requiring attentional control or not. Patients performed less well on tasks requiring attentional resources. This impairment in the use of attentional resources has a direct impact on the VTI. The Rao et al study [2] was one of the first to highlight this impairment of the VTI. In addition, some studies have pointed out that damage to the VTI is more likely to occur in relapsing-remitting and secondarily progressive forms of the disease, whereas damage to the memory of the VTI is more likely to occur in secondarily progressive forms. work would only concern secondarily progressive forms [70]. A test that essentially explores VTI: the SDMT (Symbol Digit Modalities Test). frequently impaired in MS [71]. This test is also impaired in 50% of cases from the onset of onset of the disease [72]. A deficit in the SDMT is a fairly good predictor of the onset of the disease.the existence of more global cognitive impairment [73]. The SDMT is also the best test correlated with deep grey matter atrophy [74].

Another important element in SE is working memory (WM), which appears to be affected more by a slowdown in the handling of transiently stored information than by a real capacity problem. This can be imagined by the fact that a MS patient, when he has all the time he needs to respond to performances identical to those of a healthy subject. It is therefore well established that VTI impairment, most probably linked to demyelination, is central to MS. It also contributes to deficits in other more specific cognitive functions. Cognitive impairment in MS can also have an impact on quality of life, activities and professional life. A study looking at the impact of slowing ITV on QoL and involving 52 patients with various forms of MS and varying degrees of disability was carried out. different types of disability [75], did not show an impact of ITV clearly independent of the EDSS score on QOL. However, cognitive impairment does have an impact on activity. social and professional life of MS patients [76], but also on quality of life [77].

As far as executive functions are concerned, and generally speaking, this term covers a wide range of cognitive functions such as reasoning, problem-solving, abstraction and planning, sustained attention, multi-tasking, flexibility and management of novelties, etc. These are the so-called 'high-level' functions, which are supposed to control and direct the 'lower-level' functions. These are the so-called 'high-level' functions, which are supposed to control and direct the 'lower-level' functions. They are thought to be involved in almost every aspect of human neuropsychology. Dysexecutive impairment in MS seems to be widely found [78]. Their psychometric evaluation is based on two main tests: the Stroop test and verbal fluency, particularly for relapsing-remitting forms. In BCCogSEP [79], four additional tests have been added: Direct and Indirect Digits, GoNoGo and Trail Making Test (TMT). MDT disorders also appear to be highly prevalent in MS [80], and may even be the most frequently encountered cognitive deficit [81].An MDT corresponds to a system enabling short-term maintenance and manipulation of the information required to carry out complex cognitive activities [82]. It is classically assessed by means of the digit span. It corresponds to the most a large series of items that can be retrieved immediately after presentation. Performance is first assessed in direct order (the subject has to render the items in the same order as they are presented), then in reverse order (the subject has to render the items in the same order as they are presented).(starting with the last item). A patient who presents scores of 8 and 5 digits in direct and reverse order respectively will obtain performances that remain within the norms. In neuropsychological practice, it is usual to consider the classic score of 7 items +/- 2 for the direct-order span and a value of one item ofless for the span in indirect order [83].Episodic memory impairment (EMI) is also one of the most common cognitive complaints in MS patients. The concept of EDM corresponds to the memory of events in a specific spatial and temporal context. Three processes are involved: encoding, storage and retrieval. Encoding is the phase during which the characteristics of perceptual information are processed and converted into a memory trace that can be reactivated at a later date. Storage refers to the process of reserving information for future use. The purpose of recovery is to restore the data stored during the acquisition phase.The concept of MEp also defines two components: anterograde and retrograde (which concerns memory of the distant past (autobiographical memory). It is now accepted that MS patients have a disturbed anterograde memory [84]. This major deficit has palpable consequences on patients' daily lives. The main deficit However, the exact nature of anterograde MEp deficits in MS is still debated [85]. Nevertheless, the exact nature of anterograde MEp deficits is still debated. Some studies argue for a deficit in the encoding phase, while others argue for a deficit in restitution [86].The main tools for assessing anterograde MEp are : The Grober and Buschke test [87], which is the only test that ensures that the material to be memorised has been encoded. The California Verbal Learning Test (CVLT) [88], which allows the patient to encode freely, but this test also proposes the different types of playback possible (free recall, cue recall and recognition).As for autobiographical memory, it would appear that 60% of patients suffer from it. major deficit, especially in the episodic component of autobiographical memory, while the semantic component is preserved [89].On the other hand, dementia in MS is still not clearly defined, and there is no real consensus on this. However, the multiple nature of the deficits observed is now well established. with sometimes serious consequences for daily life [90]. Approximately 20-30% of cognitively-impaired patients present with "severe dementia" [91]; the loss of autonomy linked to cognitive impairment is the main factor to be objectively assessed, which is why it is important to determine the severity of dementia. limits the frequency to around 3 to 4% of patients [92].

This is known as the dementia evolution of MS.Other clinical case series even report purely dementia in MS (without motor disability). However, these cases of dementia revealing MS are rare. As soon as a diagnosis of dementia in MS is made, it is important to better understand this dimension in order to adapt day-to-day management (adapting to the needs of the patient).home, psychological support for carers, etc.). The neuropsychological characteristics of "Dementia in MS" is compared with degenerative cortical and subcortical dementias (see table1).

Table 1: neuropsychological characteristics of cortical and subcortical dementia and "dementia in MS".

	Cortical dementia	Dementia under cortical	Dementia MS
Intellectual efficiency global	Very affected	+/- preserved	+/- preserved
Memory episodic	Very affected	Slight deficit	Very affected
Functions executive	Slight deficit	Very affected	Very affected
Bradyphrenia	+/- preserved	Very affected	Very affected
Language	Slight deficit	Preserved	Preserved
Praxis	Slight deficit	Preserved	Preserved
Gnosias	Slight deficit	Preserved	+/- preserved
Mood	+ /- preserved	Slight deficit	Slight deficit

Source: G.Defer, F.Daniel, chapter 14 (dementia). Book: multiple sclerosis: clinical and therapeutic. 2017.Elsevier Masson. B Brochet [63]

COGNITIVE EVALUATION

The tests commonly used to assess cognitive impairment in cases of suspected dementia, such as the Mini-Mental State Examination (MMSE) and the Montreal Cognitive Assessment (MOCA), are not sensitive or specific enough to assess dementia disorders. This is because other domains are usually involved in MS [30].

Various neuropsychological test batteries have been validated to assess cognitive function in MS. These include the Neuropsychological Screening Battery for Ms (NSBMS), including the Paced Auditory Serial Addition Test (PASAT) and the Brief Repeatable Battery of Neuropsychological test (BRB-N), which appeared later and were then supplemented by the SDMT [93].

A few years later, with a view to a precise neuro-psychological diagnosis, "the Minimal Assessment of Cognitive Functioning in Multiple Sclerosis (MACFIMS)" has emerged. Despite their high sensitivity, the use of these test batteries in everyday practice is complicated by the fact that they can be time-consuming to administer, but also by the fact that they can be used in a variety of ways.which may require a trained neuropsychologist. The Brief International Cognitive Assessment for Multiple Sclerosis (BICAMS) is currently being used more and more, due to its ease of administration and speed (less than 15 minutes). This validated battery is widely recommended as a tool for assessing multiple sclerosis.in MS [94].

The SDMT appears to be the most efficient diagnostic tool in the initial phases of the disease [95]. It can be administered in 05 minutes and does not require a trained neuropsychologist. The different cognitive domains measured by tests included in validated neuropsychological batteries are summarised in table 2.

Table 2: Neuropsychological tests and cognitive domains explored in MS

TESTS	Cognitive domains explored	Batteries
PASAT	VTI, working and attention memory	MS, BMS, BRB-N, MACFIMS.
SET ISAAC test	Verbal fluency	NBMS, BRB-N, MACFIM.
SDMT	VTI, attention and working memory	BRB-N, MACFIMS, BICAMS
Brief Visuospatial Memory Test- Revised	Visuospatial memory	MACIMS, BICAMS
California verbal Learning test (second edition)	Verbal learning	MACIMS, BICAMS
10/36 SPART (Spatial Recall Test)	Executive functions	BRB-N

Source: Meca-Lallana V and al [95].

A recent French consensus [96] has been drawn up with an exploration procedure neuropsychology, which deserves to be detailed in the following chapter.International recommendations emphasise the use of BICAMS. This is an assessment tool developed as a short screening battery requiring the addition of other tests.This consensus was drawn up by the "cognition" group of the SF-SEP (French-speaking MS society): http: //sfsep.org. The main aim of this "cognition" group is to update assessment tools, recommendations and publications on MS and its cognitive disorders. They have therefore selected the most relevant tests for the cognitive assessment of MS patients. To do this, a panel of experts (made up of neurologists and neuropsychologists specialising in MS) was formed. Its main objective was to propose an updated French consensual procedure for the assessment of neuropsychological support for MS patients. The members of this group met once a month for an hour and a half for a year. Their experience was defined on the basis of at least 50 patients seen per year and at least 3 years of expertise. This cognitive assessment is therefore based on the BICAMS, including the SDMT, the CVLT and the BVMT-R (Brief Visuo Spatial Memory Test Revised), which assess verbal and visual VTI and MEp respectively.Screening is carried out using the SDMT, which is a rapid test for assessing ITV, in which the patient must associate numbers with symbols presented according to a correspondence model (or key) within a limited time (90 seconds). A difference of four points in clinical studies and eight points in clinical follow-up are considered significant in both directions (improvement or worsening) [97,98]. A computerised version has has also been validated, generally on a tablet [99]. In this case, the patient answers orally and the assessor notes the correct answers on the tablet. Episodic memory, again according to the 2024 French consensus, is measured via the BICAMS by the BVMT-R (for visual memory) and the CVLT (for verbal memory) [100, 101]. These two tests provide a learning score and a delayed recall score. Recall is used to assess learning ability; and the recognition is useful for assessing storage and encoding capacities.

Short-term memory and MDT are assessed using the WAIS IV Digit Span Forward. MDT is measured by the WAIS IV Digit Span Backward [102].

The three executive functions that are essentially explored in this consensus are: mental flexibility, inhibition and verbal initiation. Flexibility can be described as the ability to move from one task to another; it can be explored by TMT A and B [103].

Inhibition is the ability to control automatic processes and resist the urge to act. sensitivity to interference. It is assessed by the Stroop test in general [104]. The GoNoGo is another tool for assessing inhibitory control, a task that also exists in the "BREF" battery. Verbal initiation refers to the ability to produce a maximum number of words in a limited time. It is tested with verbal fluency. This test can be either phonemic (words beginning with a given letter), or categorical (words in the same semantic category: cities, fruit, etc.), over a period of one or two minutes.Attentional functions include vigilance, selective attention, sustained attention and divided attention. However, these functions are highly dependent on VTI. They have have long been assessed by PASAT. During this test, the patient must add up the last two numbers heard each time, at a regular rate (2, 3 or 4 seconds) [105].

Language can be assessed by oral naming of DO-80 images [106, 107, 108]. In addition, this French cognitive study group (Jougleux C et al) also looked at psychological assessment, which remains essential because anxiety and depression are two of the most common forms of depression. symptoms common in MS. For this reason, they have favoured assessment using short scales. The Beck Depression Inventory (BDI) remains the reference scale, and a short version exists [109, 110]. The best score is 21, and a cut-off score of 7 has been defined [111]. The Hospital Anxiety and Depression Scale (HADS) is another tool for assessing depression and anxiety [112]. It is a short scale used to assess both symptoms.To conclude this French consensus, it is important to emphasise that evaluation In view of the frequency of these disorders, every patient suffering from MS should be offered cognitive and psychological treatment. This assessment should be carried out from the outset, including the

BICAMS with delayed recall for MEp tests and at least one test for each cognitive domain.This assessment should also be carried out before the introduction of immunomodulatory therapy, or within three months of its introduction [113]. Cognitive remediation could then be offered at an early stage. These experts therefore recommend that all patients should be screened at least once a year with at least one MTDS. A change of eight points would be significant and would require further evaluation [107].

In addition, another factor is increasingly incriminated in the different cognitive phenotypes of MS: this is the concept of "cognitive reserve" [114]. Patients with have a lower risk of developing cognitive disorders [115]. This reserve Cognitive ability is therefore often assessed only by IQ (intelligence quotient), without there being any real consensus on this.

Table 3 summarises all the French 2024 recommendations from the group "cognition" section of the SF-SEP.

Table 3: summary of the SF-SEP 2024 recommendations concerning the different tests to be carried out according to the cognitive domain concerned.

Cognitive domain	Specific tests
Short-term memory Working memory	Digit Span Forward and Backward (WAIS IV)
Attentional functions	PASAT 3 seconds Vigilance of the attentional performance test Shared attention to performance testing attention
Executive functions	Mental flexibility: TMT A and B, Crosstaping test (BCCogSEP), flexibility of the attentional performance test
	Verbal initiation: phonemic and categorical verbal fluency Inhibition: GoNoGo
Language	DO-80

NB: in all cases, the SDMT should be performed first.

Cognitive phenotypes have been described in a number of studies: Leavitt MV et al [116] described three cognitive phenotypes: isolated memory disorders (I), isolated slowing of the ITV (II) and combined impairment of both (III).

This study looked at 128 MS patients who underwent a full cognitive assessment, which revealed that 18.80% (phenotype I), 7.8% (phenotype II) and 17.2% (phenotype III) of the patients had the following phenotypes (phenotype III). It should be noted that 56.3% of the patients in this series had a normal cognitive assessment (see Figure 3 [116]).

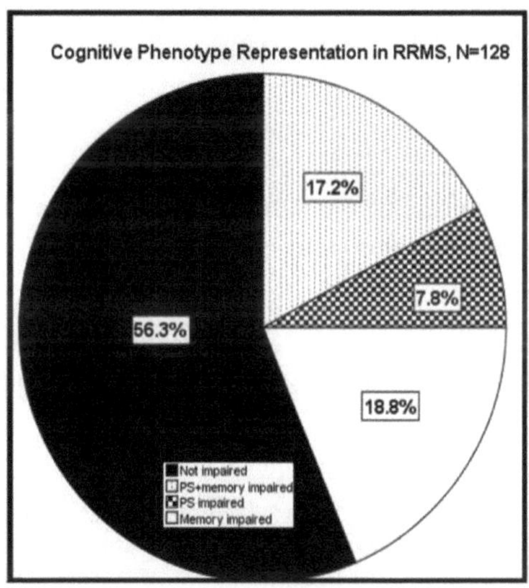

Figure 3: Percentage representation of cognitive phenotype groups in a complete sample of 128 patients with relapsing-remitting MS [114].

Another team (De Meo, E et al) [115] reported 5 cognitive phenotypes in MS:

Type I (preserved cognitive functions)
Type II (moderate impairment of verbal fluency) Type III (moderate multi-domain impairment)
Type IV (severe impairment of attention and executive functions) Type V (severe multi-domain impairment)
This is a cross-sectional study of 1212 MS patients versus 196 healthy controls.

The aim of distinguishing between these different phenotypes is to allow more accurate measurement of the phenotypes. of the cognitive state of MS patients, to support clinicians in their choice of treatment, and also to adapt cognitive remediation according to each phenotype. There are a number of clinical features worth highlighting in this study:Patients with phenotype I (preserved cognition) and those with phenotype II (moderate impairment of verbal memory and semantic fluency) have a behaviour different from the other patients. They have the same average age (around 36.5 and 38.2 years respectively) and the same duration of illness (7.3 and 7.6 years respectively). They are therefore younger and have a shorter duration of illness than the other phenotypes. (average age around 42, and duration of illness around 10 years).

- Patients with the severe multi-domain disease phenotype have motor disability

much more important than the other phenotypes (average EDSS around 3 compared with 1.5 for the moderate phenotype).
- As regards years of study, the only difference observed was between the moderate multi-domain phenotype and the phenotype with severe impairment of executive and attentional functions (12.6 years for 1[er] and 11.5 years for 2).[nd]

In this study, correlations were made between these phenotypes and imaging (see fig 4 [116]). The authors compared the population studied (the different phenotypes with each other), but also with the general population. The main conclusions were
thalamic volume is smaller in type I despite a normal cognitive work-up; cortical volume is smaller in types III, IV and V than in the general population, and in type V there is hippocampal atrophy and smaller volumes in the caudate nuclei. This study therefore enabled the identification of neuroanatomical substrates likely to explain this subdivision into cognitive phenotypes.

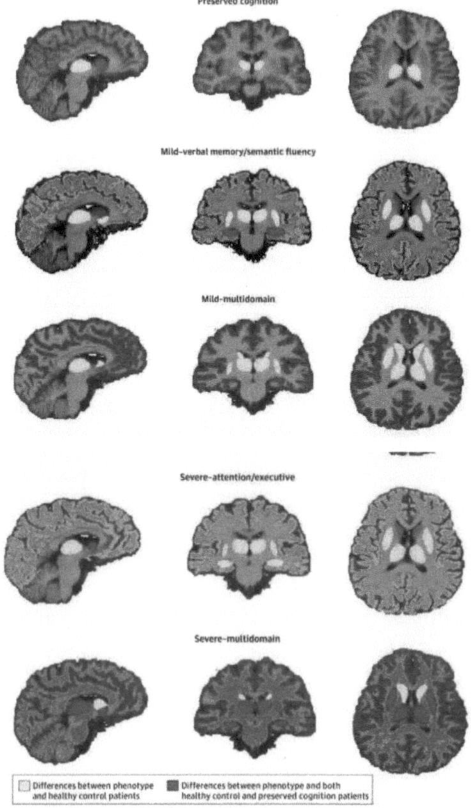

Figure 4: Magnetic resonance imaging characteristics of cognitive phenotypes [116].

This cross-sectional study therefore made it possible to distinguish different cognitive phenotypes in a large cohort of MS patients, as well as to characterise certain cognitive features of the disease. radiological correlations with MRI. Nevertheless, these phenotypes can be represented as a continuum, and it can sometimes be difficult to differentiate between them.

Phenotype I (preserved cognition) seems to prevail in the early stages of the disease, with a shorter duration of illness and a smaller thalamic volume than in individuals healthy.

Phenotype II (mild impairment of verbal memory / semantic fluency) is characterised by

by hippocampal atrophy, which appears to be a potential pathological substrate. Hippocampal lesions in T2 hypersignal with the phenomenon of dysconnectivity engendered by the hippocampal atrophy.
also appear to be associated with this phenotype.

Phenotype III (moderate multi-domain involvement) has cortical atrophy as a distinctive MRI feature.
Phenotype IV (severe executive and attentional impairment) is characterised by a reduction in performance on all tests, with a significant lesion load in the white matter near the ventricles. This radiological aspect is also associated with higher levels of fatigue in MS patients [117].
Phenotype V (severe multi-domain disease) is characterised by a significant reduction in performance on cognitive tests. This phenotype appears to be more common in advanced stages of the disease. of MS, but it is also found in newly diagnosed patients and could be considered a poor prognostic factor at this stage. These patients also showed severe brain atrophy on MRI, as well as an association with symptoms of severe depression [118, 119].
This new categorisation of cognitive deficits could integrate the EDSS score in the definition of clinical disability, in order to assist practitioners in their therapeutic choices and help them adapt cognitive rehabilitation strategies.

COGNITION SOCIAL

Among the cognitive dysfunctions observed in people with MS, it has been reported that they affect not only perceptual-motor functions, but also language, memory and memory working memory, sustained attention, speed of information processing, and the ability to executive functions, but also CS [120]. EC encompasses the mental operations that underlie social interactions, in particular the ability to perceive, interpret and react to the intentions, dispositions and behaviours of others. This definition makes it possible to It can be distinguished from broader cognitive functions such as memory, attention and executive functions, which are generally affected by cognitive disorders [121]. CS is a neurocognitive capacity, which includes different aspects of processing, decision-making or responding to the demands of social stimuli and can affect various disorders neurological [122]. The key components of CS include theory of mind (the ability to attribute mental states to oneself and to others), recognition of emotions (the ability to identify and respond to emotional expressions), empathy (the ability to understand and share the feelings of others) and social perception (the ability to identify and respond to the feelings of others).ability to decode social cues and contexts) [123]. These cognitive processes are essential for effective communication and social functioning, and impairments in CS can have a significant impact on quality of life and interactions. people suffering from neurological disorders.Quality of life is a broad, multidimensional concept that generally includes subjective assessments of both positive and negative aspects of life. For people with chronic diseases such as multiple sclerosis, quality of life encompasses health physical condition, psychological state, level of independence, social relationships, personal beliefs and relationships with significant elements of their environment [124]. Impaired CS has a significant impact on quality of life. Impairments in CS are important predictors of reduced quality of life in MS because they result in impairment of the activities of daily living and are independent of motor disability. However, the authors of various studies suggest that cognitive decline has an impact on both CS and quality of life [125].

Although some studies have explored the potential link between quality of life and CS, much of the research remains unclear. There is therefore an urgent need to focus on assessment of CS, particularly in the early stages of MS, to better understand its impact on quality of life and develop interventions to improve patient outcomes. However, it is very difficult to isolate one element (such as social cognition) and estimate its impact on the quality of life of multiple sclerosis patients. This difficulty is due to the fact that many many elements are present in the disease and that they are closely linked. Adequate social support has been associated with better quality of life, including improved psychological well-being and better disease management [126]. By Consequently, interventions aimed at strengthening social support networks can play a crucial role in optimising the quality of life of people living with MS. At

In short, MS poses multifaceted challenges that go beyond physical symptoms and encompass cognitive, emotional and social dimensions. It is essential to recognise and take into account these various aspects of the disease in order to improve overall results and quality of life for people affected by this doubly disabling condition.

CLINICAL-RADIOLOGICAL CORRELATIONS

MRI is an extremely sensitive radiological examination for the detection of abnormalities.specific to MS. Various techniques have been validated for its exploration, such as T1, T2, T2* and flair sequences. The emergence of these techniques to define MRI structural correlates with cognitive impairment in MS have been studied in different cohorts of patients; these studies have showed lesions which may be diffuse or focal in the grey matter [127, 128], with, in particular, diffuse microstructural anomalies [129, 130] or even irreversible tissue loss [131]. All these radiological aspects seem to play an important role in the presence and severity of cognitive disorders [132]. In an Italian work (Preziosa. P et al. 2016) [130], atrophy of different regions affecting both white matter and grey matter is linked to reduced performance in different cognitive domains (figure 5 [130]). No correlation has been found between regional atrophy affecting the grey matter and verbal memory, as well as atrophied regions of the white matter with verbal memory and fluency. In fact, before any global deficit in MS, diffusion anomalies in the white matter and atrophy of certain critical regions of the grey matter lead to mediocre cognitive performance in this cohort; this is due to probably due to a disconnection syndrome occurring between regions of grey matter and lesions of white matter. Conversely, the alteration of certain areas was associated with structural lesions in certain regions that may play a critical role in the cognitive function studied. This being the case, the use of the usual MRI sequences may not be sufficient to make correct radio-cognitive correlations.

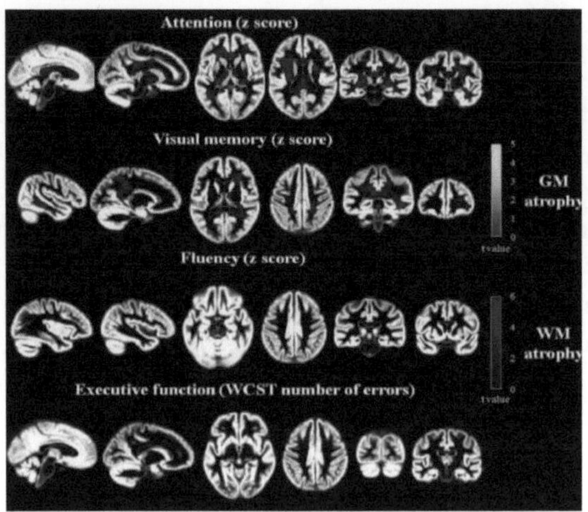

Figure 5: Statistical parametric mapping (SPM) analysis showing the regions with grey matter (GM) atrophy (coded yellow) and white matter (WM) atrophy (coded blue) in patients with multiple sclerosis, significantly correlated with performance in different cognitive domains (Source: [130]).

The severity of cognitive deficits in MS differs according to its clinical form. It is assumed that this cognitive dysfunction is already present in the early stages of the disease (CIS or RIS), and that it progresses in parallel with the accumulation of disability [133]. The data currently available suggest that cognitive decline is more severe in progressive forms of the disease [134].

In some series of patients with the RR form and a disease duration of more than 10 years, the results of certain psychomotor tests (the numerical digit span test and SDMT) indicated that these patients were deficient; whereas patients with an early progressive form obtained results below the normal in all neuropsychological tests. However, no significant difference was observed between secondarily progressive forms (SP) and primary progressive forms (pp) [135]. In a large Italian cohort of 1040 patients [133], the prevalence of CT was 46.3%. This proportion was subdivided according to the progressive forms of the disease: 34.5 in CIS patients, 44.5% in patients with relapsing-remitting disease, 79.4% in patients with relapsing-remitting disease. patients with a secondarily progressive form and 91.3% of patients with a PP form. VTI was the cognitive domain most frequently found in all the groups in this study. It should be noted that a significant difference was observed between relapsing-remitting and progressive forms, but not between CIS and RR forms, or between SP and PP forms.A meta-analysis of 47 series (4,460 patients) showed that patients with progressive forms had moderately more severe deficits in cognitive domains than RR forms, with notable differences in verbal learning, VTI and verbal memory [134]. A greater lesion load and more severe disability, as well as the role of neurodegeneration and cerebral atrophy, seem to explain this difference [136].

FACTORS INFLUENCING COGNITIVE FUNCTION IN SEPSIS

Several factors are known to influence the level of cognitive dysfunction. Regular physical exercise, absence of addictions, a healthy diet and control of certain comorbidities can have a positive effect on cognition in MS patients [136]. There is also increasing evidence that early initiation of RRMS-specific disease-modifying therapy can stabilise or even improve cognition [137].

In the COGIMUS study [138], cognitive decline was reduced by 32% in patients treated with interferon B 44 ug 3 times a week for at least 03 years. Another treatment (Natalizumab) has also been shown to be effective for TC, depression and fatigue [139].

It is important to note that the drugs traditionally used in certain degenerative dementias have been shown to be ineffective in MS patients [140]. Psychiatric disorders are also thought to influence the cognitive abilities of MS patients. These include depression, which affects about 30% of patients [141].

Several studies have revealed a negative impact of depressive symptoms on cognitive functions, in particular VTI, executive functions, attention and memory [142]. Anxiety disorders, which affect around 22% of MS patients [143], mainly influence executive functions and episodic memory. Another factor that can influence cognitive problems is fatigue, which affects up to 80% of MS patients [144] and is defined by patients as general tiredness or lassitude. even without physical effort. One of its components is cognitive fatigue, defined as a reduction in performance on tasks involving continuous cognitive effort [145].The effect of vitamin D supplementation on cognition has also been discussed. It could be beneficial in people with low levels of vitamin D or a lower cognitive functioning. It essentially improves non-verbal memory [146].

COGNITIVE GROWTH

An MS relapse is defined as a new, worsened or worsening neurological symptom. relapsing, corresponding to disease activity and/or acute MRI lesions, occurring at least 30 days after the onset of a previous symptom and lasting at least 24 hours, in the absence of fever or infection. Clinically, relapse is confirmed when symptoms are accompanied by an objective neurological change compared with the state of previous stable clinical state, as determined by assessment of the EDSS. Acute MRI lesions may or may not be accompanied by clinical symptoms, as the activity Neuroinflammation does not always lead to a flare-up or clinical symptoms. This silent activity of MS without any visible clinical manifestation is at the heart of the NEDA concept or "absence of evidence of disease activity" [147, 148]. This NEDA concept is essentially used to improve the prognosis of MS and optimise treatment of the disease. It consists of three criteria: absence of relapses, absence of progression of the disability and absence of activity on MRI (new or enlarged T2 lesions or T1 gadolinium-enhanced images, which may recur [149]. However, it is quite difficult to determine whether this is a cognitive relapse in an MS patient with a change in mental status or in a patient with cognitive dysfunction and signs of relapse on MRI, but without clinical signs of acute disease activity. Recent studies have identified the neuropsychological phenotype of MS patients with cognitive decline and which could be identified by the SDMT. Monitoring decline before and during the relapse period, could allow a significant change in the SDMT score to be observed. A change in the SDMT score of 4 points or a change of 10% is considered significant, as discussed above (test chapters). neuropsychological tests). Prospective studies assessing cognitive impairment using SDMT, in patients with relapsing MS and controls, distinguished the two groups, during a relapse, by 5 SDMT points. Several months later, the difference was reduced to 3 SDMT points. These results indicate that it is possible to identify MS patients showing cognitive changes in the context of a relapse, using the SDMT [150]. The results of these studies showed that changes in the SDMT were greater in relapsing patients, and that SDMT could be considered a significant tool for detecting cognitive relapse [151]. In addition, SDMT correlates well with MRI parameters of cerebral atrophy (loss of grey matter, etc.).cortical and third ventricle with or thalamic and hypothalamic fraction) [152], so that measurement of cortical thickness correlates well with cognitive tests in MS [153, 154]. Lesions located in the frontal and mesial temporal lobes and in the medulla oblongata are associated with cognitive deficit and fatigue. Lesions located in the deep grey matter of the thalamus and hypothalamus correlate with deficits in visuo-spatial memory and reduced information processing speed [155, 156].

THE IMPACT OF COGNITIVE IMPAIRMENT ON PATIENTS AND THEIR CARERS

Research shows that cognitive problems associated with MS are significantly associated with significant to poor health-related quality of life, including difficulties in activities of daily living, social and professional life, and family relationships [157]. Impaired cognitive function has a greater effect on employment than physical disability, such as losing a job due to poor performance [5]. Despite the importance of cognitive impairment in the daily functioning of people with MS and the fact that approximately 80% of people with MS live with family members [158], little research has examined the impact of cognitive changes on close relationships with informal carers. Several studies have explored the impact of a partner's MS diagnosis on the couple's relationship, including strategies adaptation techniques used [159]. Communication problems have received particular attention. One study found that direct caregivers of people with MS reported relationship problems such as loss of intimacy and reduced communication due to the partner's reduced cognitive capacity [160].

An American study [161] was based on individual telephone interviews with 30 participants (15 adults with MS and their 15 spouses/partners). In contacting the research team, potential participants were assessed for determine the willingness of their spouse or partner living at home who is their main carer to participate, and also access to a telephone and the Internet (computer laptop, tablet or smartphone) in a private setting. Topics covered included the impact of cognitive difficulties on themselves and their partners and on their social relationships, their perceived need and desire for help and support, and the desired outcomes associated with this help. The impact could vary from one patient to another, sometimes with several of them that can be observed in the same patient. A significant social impact has been noted, which may relate to a feeling of lack of support from family and friends, a feeling of isolation from family and friends, and a feeling of isolation from friends. feelings of isolation, as well as difficulties in managing various social events. A 2^e observed impact is the changes that can affect daily life, in particular a change in abilities prior to the illness, with emotional reactions. which may be exaggerated, and job loss, especially if the work is intellectual in nature. A 3^e impact noted concerning the quality of the relationship with one's spouse, which may be deteriorating.

Nevertheless, the impact of cognitive impairment on both the person with MS and their partner, including health-related quality of life, communication, quality of relationships and performance of daily activities, can be improved by encouragingpositive coping strategies. The partner plays a major role in helping the person with MS adapt to cognitive problems, and it is important that practitioners provide information and resources to the family at the time of diagnosis and direct them to the relevant agencies for further support. In this study, participants expressed a desire for more support, such as education on strategies for overcoming common challenges in communication and activities of daily living.

MANAGEMENT OF COGNITIVE DISORDERS IN SEPSIS

To date, there is no symptomatic treatment for cognitive difficulties in MS or other neurological diseases. Cognitive rehabilitation remains a good therapeutic tool for improving or maintaining good cognitive function. However, the treatment of these cognitive disorders is based on three pillars: pharmacological treatment, symptomatic treatment and cognitive rehabilitation.

1 -Pharmacological treatment :

Over the last 20 years, a wide range of treatments has been made available to people with MS. In principle, these DMTs (Disease Modifiying therapies) have the potential to positively influence cognitive outcomes by acting on mechanisms key pathogens underlying MS-related cognitive impairment [162].

To date, no significant efficacy has been observed when using specific MS treatments. DMTs such as interferons Beta1a and Beta1b, deacetylcholine glatiramer, natalizumab, teriflunomide, fingolimod and ocrelizumab can affect disease activity (relapse rate) and in some cases the progression of disability. These drugs could have a positive impact on the long-term cognitive outcome of a people with MS. In fact, all treatments reduce the accumulation of irreversible lesions in the nervous system, with positive effects on the T2 cerebral lesion load, as well as sometimes reducing cerebral atrophy. In this context, so-called "high efficacy" DMTs such as Natalizumab (NTZ) and Rituximab appear to have a greater effect than so-called 1^e line therapies [163]. The data suggest that high efficacy therapies should be more effective in preserving cognitive function as higher rates of cortical volume loss have been associated with greater cognitive decline. important [164]. Unfortunately, the data that could confirm this are scarce. Many gaps remain due to a methodology that is not unified between the different series, and follow-up times are still too short. However, as mentioned above, most clinical studies have not found a spectacular effect on cognition, with the possible exception of natalizumab [165].
However, all the pivotal studies carried out on DMTs up to 2023 have produced positive results. mixed results, probably due to the short duration of the trials and/or problems methodology. The recommended inclusion of SDMT as an outcome measure in future trials could provide additional insight [166].

A relatively recent meta-analysis (Landmeyer et al.) [167] evaluated different DMTs on performance in cognitive tests in adults with relapsing MS: 44 eligible studies were then analysed in this work. All these studies evaluated the effects of at least one DMT and reported positive effects on at least one cognitive test, evaluated at baseline and during follow-up. These effects were essentially limited to VTI measured by the SDMT or PASAT. However, these studies involved patient populations that were heterogeneous, with variable evaluation tools and variable criteria. Furthermore, this meta-analysis did not reveal any superior effects of therapeutic escalation on cognition. However, a recent study presented at the International Congress on MS (ECTRIMS/ACTRIMS: European and American committee for treatment and research in multiple sclerosis) in October 2023 in Milan, Italy, proved that DMTs could improve cognitive function in MS [168]. This was demonstrated by comparing treated versus untreated patients. This study was conducted on more than 11,000 patients, recruited from 10 centres in three countries. This study included all treatments known today, whether platform therapies or highly effective treatments. The effects were comparable in both groups. However, another study, from Sweden, looked at NTZ and compared its efficacy with that of other treatments. with other DMTs [169]. The data were collected from the rich Swedish register of MS patients over a period from 2007 to 2020. An increase in SDMT score of more than 10%, compared with the baseline value, was defined as a cognitive improvement. This probability of improvement was compared between the people treated with NTZ and those treated with other DMTs. 2100 patients on NTZ were included and 2622 on other DMTs. At six months' follow-up, 45% of patients reported improvement, with better results in the NTZ group. The chances of improvement increased by 7% per month of NTZ treatment, compared with 4% for the other groups. monoclonal antibodies; and it was not significant for platform therapies. This study therefore highlights the fact that treatment with NTZ or other monoclonal antibodies is associated with a significantly faster probability of cognitive improvement than platform therapies.

2 - Symptomatic treatment :

The importance of these treatments has often been emphasised in studies, but unfortunately the results have been negative or inconsistent in terms of CT.
Acting on fatigue with drugs such as amantadine, modafinil, etc. depression and anxiety with psychostimulants and antidepressants, and specific treatments for Alzheimer's disease are still therapeutic options. promising, but still insufficient [170].

3 - Cognitive remediation (CR):

This is a non-pharmacological approach, the aim of which is to maintain good cognitive function by improving it through training, exercises, and methods of compensation and adaptation designed to optimise residual cognitive function as far as possible. These cognitive remediation techniques have two main aims: an effect on brain activation, proven by functional imaging [171], and a clinical effect on memory [172].

The aim of this management is to reduce the impact of cognitive impairment on the The aim is to help patients regain their functional autonomy, with a view to improving their quality of life. These rehabilitation methods involve several group workshops, in which one function is worked on at each meeting. The results are very positive. encouraging results [173]. In other words, CR can be conceptualised as a process by which the people with brain injuries work with healthcare professionals to remedy or alleviate cognitive deficits resulting from neurological damage [174]. It encompasses a wide range of behavioural therapeutic interventions based on clinical neuropsychology and behavioural analysis, cognitive retraining, individual and group psychotherapy, and the concepts of neuroplasticity and reserve. cognitive [175].

In clinical practice, this CR is based on the person, whose aim is essentially to improve quality of life. The aim of these interventions may be compensatory, i.e. to help patients adapt to their cognitive problems, or restorative, i.e. to reinforce or improve the deficient cognitive areas that are causing a disability with repercussions on life. or a combination of the two [176]. All these forms of cognitive rehabilitation are presumed to function at the neurobiological level via the neuroplasticity (brain activation and increased functional connectivity). Concomitant management of other comorbidities (depression, fatigue, anxiety) is essential in order to optimise CR therapy. Step 1^e involves identifying and defining the nature of the impaired cognitive domain and providing initial psycho-education. Step 2nde involves choosing between the most effective cognitive rehabilitation intervention options, and adapting them to each patient. These so-called"Compensatory" drugs appear to be effective in people with mild to moderate attention and memory difficulties [177]. A recent meta-analysis [178] reviewed all blinded randomised controlled trials in adults with MS published between 2013 and 2021. A final list of 26 studies was selected. Three main categories of attitude stand out: specific individual rehabilitation, group rehabilitation and computer-based training. Among the individualised studies, five were devoted to memory, while the others covered several cognitive domains.The overall results of all these studies support the efficacy of CR, as assessed by objective improvement in neuropsychological tests. Artificial intelligence algorithms now make it possible to obtain an increasingly detailed cognitive profile of the MS patient [179]. Remote cognitive rehabilitation techniques make it possible to improve the personalisation of the various CR interventions. Furthermore, an increasing number of studies are highlighting the notion of selecting or even triaging patients who may benefit most from CR [180, 181]. The CRAMMS (Cognitive Rehabilitation for Attention and Memory in MS) study demonstrated the efficacy of RC in improving cognitive function, but in some patients more than others. The results extracted from this study suggest that younger participants with an average to high level of education, diagnosed with relapsing-remitting and primary-progressive MS, with no recent relapses, and with mild to moderate cognitive difficulties, are the most likely to benefit from CR. These evolutionary predictions therefore make it possible to optimise the resources that may be limited in order to provide optimum CR for the most sensitive subjects.

CONCLUSION

MS-related CTs appear to be becoming very frequent, early onset and disabling. They should be assessed as early as possible. Different cognitive profiles are increasingly being reported. Characterising them would enable optimal management and recovery. better. Medicinal management is becoming increasingly clear, and appears to be positive with monoclonal antibodies, compared with platform therapies, which nevertheless retain a partial benefit. CR workshops seem to be a good non-drug alternative, to be adapted to the cognitive profile identified, taking into account the epidemiological factors favourable to a better therapeutic response, factors which are now beginning to be well understood. individualised.

REFERENCES

1. Amato MP, Portaccio E, Goretti B, Zipoli V, Hakiki B, Giannini M, Pastò L, Razzolini L. Cognitive impairment in early stages of multiple sclerosis. Neurol Sci. 2010 Nov;31(Suppl 2):S211-4. doi: 10.1007/s10072-010-0376-4.

2. Rao SM, Leo GJ, Bernardin L, Unverzagt F. Cognitive dysfunction in multiple sclerosis. I. Frequency, patterns, and prediction. Neurology. 1991 May;41(5):685-91. doi: 10.1212/wnl.41.5.685.

3. Rao SM. Neuropsychology of multiple sclerosis. Curr Opin Neurol. 1995 Jun;8(3):216-20. doi: 10.1097/00019052-199506000-00010.

4. Amato MP, Zipoli V, Portaccio E. Cognitive changes in multiple sclerosis. Expert Rev Neurother. 2008 Oct;8(10):1585-96. doi: 10.1586/14737175.8.10.1585.

5. Chiaravalloti ND, DeLuca J. Cognitive impairment in multiple sclerosis. Lancet Neurol. 2008 Dec;7(12):1139-51. doi: 10.1016/S1474-4422(08)70259-X.

6. Amato MP, Hakiki B, Goretti B, Rossi F, Stromillo ML, Giorgio A, Roscio M, Ghezzi A, Guidi L, Bartolozzi ML, Portaccio E, De Stefano N; Italian RIS/MS Study Group. Association of MRI metrics and cognitive impairment in radiologically isolated syndromes. Neurology. 2012 Jan 31;78(5):309-14. doi: 10.1212/WNL.0b013e31824528c9.

7. Zipoli V, Goretti B, Hakiki B, Siracusa G, Sorbi S, Portaccio E, Amato MP. Cognitive impairment predicts conversion to multiple sclerosis in clinically isolated syndromes. Mult Scler. 2010 Jan;16(1):62-7. doi: 10.1177/1352458509350311.

8. Benedict RHB, Amato MP, DeLuca J, Geurts JJG. Cognitive impairment in multiple sclerosis: clinical management, MRI, and therapeutic avenues. Lancet Neurol. 2020 Oct;19(10):860-871. doi: 10.1016/S1474-4422(20)30277-5.

9. Rao SM. A manual for the brief repeatable battery of neuropsychological tests in multiple sclerosis. Milwaukee Med Coll Wis 1990;1696.

10. Dujardin K, Sockeel P, Cabaret M, De Seze J, Vermersch P. [BCcogSEP: a French test battery evaluating cognitive functions in multiple sclerosis]. Rev Neurol (Paris) 2004; 160:51-62.

11. Goverover Y, Genova H, Hillary F, DeLuca J. The relationship between

neuropsychological measures and the Timed Instrumental Activities of Daily Living task in multiple sclerosis. Mult Scler 2007 ;13:636-44. http://dx.doi.org/ 10.1177/1352458506072984

12. Mitchell AJ, Benito-Leon J, Gonzalez J-MM, Rivera-Navarro J. Quality of life and its assessment in multiple sclerosis: integrating physical and psychological components of wellbeing. Lancet Neurol 2005; 4:556-66

13. Weld-Blundell IV, Grech L, Learmonth YC, Marck CH. Lifestyle and complementary therapies in multiple sclerosis guidelines: systematic review. Acta Neurol Scand 2022;145:379-92. http://dx.doi.org/10.1111/ane.13574

14. Brissart H, Omorou AY, Forthoffer N, Berger E, Moreau T, De Seze J, et al. Memory improvement in multiple sclerosis after an extensive cognitive rehabilitation program in groups with a multicenter double-blind randomized trial. Clin Rehabil 2020;34:754-63. http://dx.doi.org/10.1177/ 0269215520920333.

15. Zipoli V, Goretti B, Hakiki B, Siracusa G, Sorbi S, Portaccio E, et al. Cognitive impairment predicts conversion to multiple sclerosis in clinically isolated syndromes. Mult Scler 2009;16:62-7. http://dx.doi.org/10.1177/1352458509350311

16. Cheng EM, Crandall CJ, Bever CT, Giesser B, Haselkorn JK, Hays RD, et al. Quality indicators for multiple sclerosis. Mult Scler 2010;16:970-80. http://dx.doi.org/10.1177/ 1352458510372394.

17. Olek, M.J. Multiple Sclerosis. Ann. Intern. Med. 2021, 174, ITC81-ITC96
18. Frith, C.D. Social Cognition. Philos. Trans. R. Soc. B Biol. Sci. 2008, 363, 2033-2039.
19. McIntosh-Michaelis SA, Roberts MH, WilkinsonSM, Diamond ID, McLellan DL, Martin JP, et al. The prevalence of cognitive impairment in a community survey of multiple sclerosis. Br J Clin Psychol 1991; 30 : 333-48

20. Deloire MS, Bonnet MC, Salort E, Arimone Y, Boudineau M, Petry KG, Brochet B. How to detect cognitive dysfunction at early stages of multiple sclerosis? Mult Scler. 2006 Aug;12(4):445-52. doi: 10.1191/1352458506ms1289oa.

21. Kediha Mi, Boulekouiret S, Hecham N, Nouioua S, Ali Pacha L. Cognitive impairment in clinically isolated syndromes: A control-case study. Journal de la faculté de médecine d'Oran. 2020 Jun 21;4(1):547-52.

22. Pitteri M, Romualdi C, Magliozzi Ret al. Cognitive impairment predicts

disability progression and cortical thining in MS: an 8-year study. Mult Scler 2017;23(6):848-854. doi:10.1177/1352458516665496

23. Van Schependom J, D'hooghe MB, Cleynhens K, D'hooge M, Haelewyck MC, De Keyser J, Nagels G. The Symbol Digit Modalities Test as sentinel test for cognitive impairment in multiple sclerosis. Eur J Neurol. 2014 Sep;21(9):1219-25, e71-2. doi: 10.1111/ene.12463.

24. Zakzanis KK. Distinct neurocognitive profiles in multiple sclerosis subtypes. Arch Clin Neuropsychol. 2000 Feb;15(2):115-36.

25. Achiron A, Chapman J, Magalashvili D, Dolev M, Lavie M, Bercovich E, Polliack M, Doniger GM, Stern Y, Khilkevich O, Menascu S, Hararai G, Gurevich M, Barak Y. Modeling of cognitive impairment by disease duration in multiple sclerosis: a cross-sectional study. PLoS One. 2013 Aug 1;8(8):e71058. doi: 10.1371/journal.pone.0071058.

26. Moccia M, Lanzillo R, Palladino R, Chang KC, Costabile T, Russo C, De Rosa A, Carotenuto A, Saccà F, Maniscalco GT, Brescia Morra V. Cognitive impairment at diagnosis predicts 10-year multiple sclerosis progression. Mult Scler. 2016 Apr;22(5):659-67. doi: 10.1177/1352458515599075.

27. Dorstyn DS, Roberts RM, Murphy G, Haub R. Employment and multiple sclerosis: A meta-analytic review of psychological correlates. J Health Psychol. 2019 Jan;24(1):38-51. doi: 10.1177/1359105317691587.

28. Strober LB, Callanan RM. Unemployment in multiple sclerosis across the ages: How factors of unemployment differ among the decades of life. J Health Psychol. 2021 Aug;26(9):1353-1363. doi: 10.1177/1359105319876340.

29. Migliore S, Ghazaryan A, Simonelli I, Pasqualetti P, Squitieri F, Curcio G, Landi D, Palmieri MG, Moffa F, Filippi MM, Vernieri F. Cognitive Impairment in Relapsing-Remitting Multiple Sclerosis Patients with Very Mild Clinical Disability. Behav Neurol. 2017;2017:7404289. doi: 10.1155/2017/7404289.

30. McNicholas N, O'Connell K, Yap SM, Killeen RP, Hutchinson M, McGuigan C. Cognitive dysfunction in early multiple sclerosis: a review. QJM. 2018 Jun 1;111(6):359-364. doi: 10.1093/qjmed/hcx070.

31. Langdon D: Cognitive impairment in multiple sclerosisrecent advances and future prospects. Eur Neurol Rev 2010; 5: 69±72. doi: http : //dx.doi.org/ 10.17925/enr.2010.05.01.69

32. Strober L, Englert J, Munschauer F, Weinstock-Guttman B, Rao S, Benedict

RH. Sensitivity of conventional memory tests in multiple sclerosis: comparing the Rao Brief Repeatable Neuropsychological Battery and the Minimal Assessment of Cognitive Function in MS. Mult Scler. 2009;15(9):1077-1084. doi:10.1177/1352458509106615

33. Kalmar JH, Gaudino EA, Moore NB, Halper J, Deluca J. The relationship between cognitive deficits and everyday functional activities in multiple sclerosis. Neuropsychology 2008; 22:442-449. doi:10.1037/0894-4105.22.4.442

34. Sumowski, J.F.; Benedict, R.; Enzinger, C.; Filippi, M.; Geurts, J.J.; Hamalainen, P.; Hulst, H.; Inglese, M.; Leavitt, V.M.; Rocca, M.A.; et al. Cognition in multiple sclerosis, State of the field and priorities for the future. Neurology 2018, 90, 278-288.

35. Raggi, A.; Covelli, V.; Schiavolin, S.; Scaratti, C.; Leonardi, M.; Willems, M. Work-related problems in multiple sclerosis: A literature review on its associates and determinants. Disabil. Rehabil. 2016, 38, 936-944.

36. Schiavolin, S.; Leonardi, M.; Giovannetti, A.M.; Antozzi, C.; Brambilla, L.; Confalonieri, P.;Mantegazza, R.; Raggi, A. Factors related to difficulties with employment in patients with multiple sclerosis: A review of 2002-2011 literature. Int. J. Rehabil. Res. 2013, 36, 105-111.

37. Mickens, M.N.; Perrin, P.B.; Aguayo, A.; Rabago, B.; Macias-Islas, M.; Arango-Lasprilla, J.

Mediational Model of Multiple Sclerosis Impairments, Family Needs, and Caregiver Mental Health in Guadalajara, Mexico. Behav. Neurol. 2018

38. Eijlers AJC, van Geest Q, Dekker I, Steenwijk MD, Meijer KA, Hulst HE, Barkhof F, Uitdehaag BMJ, Schoonheim MM, Geurts JJG. Predicting cognitive decline in multiple sclerosis: a 5-year follow-up study. Brain. 2018 Sep 1;141(9):2605-2618. doi: 10.1093/brain/awy202. PMID: 30169585.

39. Gaetani L, Salvadori N, Chipi E, Gentili L, Borrelli A, Parnetti L, Di Filippo M. Cognitive impairment in multiple sclerosis: lessons from cerebrospinal fluid biomarkers. Neural Regen Res. 2021 Jan;16(1):36-42. doi: 10.4103/1673-5374.286949.

40. Preziosa P, Pagani E, Meani A, Storelli L, Margoni M, Yudin Y, Tedone N, Biondi D, Rubin M, Rocca MA, Filippi M. Chronic Active Lesions and Larger Choroid Plexus Explain Cognition and Fatigue in Multiple Sclerosis. Neurol Neuroimmunol Neuroinflamm. 2024 Mar;11(2):e200205. doi:

10.1212/NXI.0000000000200205.

41. Rocca MA, Amato MP, De Stefano N, et al. Clinical and imaging assessment of cognitive dysfunction in multiple sclerosis. Lancet Neurol. 2015;14(3):302-317. doi: 10.1016/S1474-4422(14)70250-9

42. Marchesi O, Vizzino C, Filippi M, Rocca MA. Current perspectives on the diagnosis and management of fatigue in multiple sclerosis. Expert Rev Neurother. 2022;22(8): 681-693. doi:10.1080/14737175.2022.2106854

43. Mesaros S, Rocca MA, Kacar K, et al. Diffusion tensor MRI tractography and cognitive impairment in multiple sclerosis. Neurology. 2012;78(13):969-975. doi:10.1212/ WNL.0b013e31824d5859

44. Preziosa P, Pagani E, Meani A, et al. NODDI, diffusion tensor microstructural abnormalities and atrophy of brain white matter and gray matter contribute to cognitive impairment in multiple sclerosis. J Neurol. 2023;270(2):810-823. doi:10.1007/ s00415-022-11415-1

45. Dal-Bianco A, Grabner G, Kronnerwetter C, et al. Long-term evolution of multiple sclerosis iron rim lesions in 7 T MRI. Brain. 2021;144(3):833-847. doi:10.1093/ brain/awaa436

46. Ghersi-Egea JF, Strazielle N, Catala M, Silva-Vargas V, Doetsch F, Engelhardt B. Molecular anatomy and functions of the choroidal blood-cerebrospinal fluid barrier in health and disease. Acta Neuropathol. 2018;135(3):337-361. doi:10.1007/s00401- 018-1807-1

47. Bergsland N, Dwyer MG, Jakimovski D, et al. Association of choroid plexus inflammation on MRI with clinical disability progression over 5 years in patients with multiple sclerosis. Neurology. 2023;100(9):e911-e920. doi:10.1212/WNL.0000000000201608

48. Mahad DH, Trapp BD, Lassmann H. Pathological mechanisms in progressive multiple sclerosis. Lancet Neurol. 2015;14(2):183-193. doi:10.1016/S1474-4422(14) 70256-X

49. Marcille M, Hurtado Rua S, Tyshkov C, et al. Disease correlates of rim lesions on quantitative

susceptibility mapping in multiple sclerosis. Sci Rep. 2022;12(1):4411. doi:10.1038/s41598-022-08477- 6

50. Absinta M, Sati P, Masuzzo F, et al. Association of chronic active multiple sclerosis lesions with disability in vivo. JAMA Neurol. 2019;76(12):1474-1483.

doi:10.1001/ jamaneurol.2019.2399

51. V.A.G. Ricigliano, B. Stankoff, Implication physiopathologique des plexus choroïdes dans la sclérose en plaques,Pratique Neurologique - FMC, Volume 15, Issue 1, 2024, Pages 67-70, ISSN 1878-7762, https://doi.org/10.1016/j.praneu.2024.01.001.

52. Bergsland N,Dwyer MG,Jakimovski D,et al.Association of choroid plexus inflammation on MRI with clinical disability progression over 5 years in patients with multiple sclerosis. Neurology.2023;100(9):e911-e920.doi:10.1212/WNL.0000000000201608

53. Wang X,Zhu Q,Yan Z,et al.Enlarged choroid plexus related to iron rim lesions and deep gray matter atrophy in relapsing-remitting multiple sclerosis.Mult Scler Relat Disord.2023;75:104740.doi:10.1016/j.msard.2023.104740

54. Rodriguez-Lorenzo S, Konings J, van der Pol S, et al. Inflammation of the choroid plexus in progressive multiple sclerosis: accumulation of granulocytes and T cells. Acta Neuropathol Commun. 2020;8(1):9. doi:10.1186/s40478-020-0885-1

55. Ruano L, Portaccio E, Goretti B, et al. Age and disability drive cognitive impairment in multiple sclerosis across disease subtypes. Mult Scler 2017; 23: 1258-67

56. Gentile A, Mori F, Bernardini S, Centonze D. Role of amyloid-β CSF levels in cognitive deficit in MS. Clin Chim Acta. 2015 Sep 20;449:23-30. doi: 10.1016/j.cca.2015.01.035.

57. Di Filippo M, Portaccio E, Mancini A, Calabresi P. Multiple sclerosis and cognition: synaptic failure and network dysfunction. Nat Rev Neurosci. 2018 Oct;19(10):599-609. doi: 10.1038/s41583-018-0053- 9.

58. Gaetani L, Blennow K, Calabresi P, Di Filippo M, Parnetti L, Zetterberg H. Neurofilament light chain as a biomarker in neurological disorders. J Neurol Neurosurg Psychiatry. 2019 Aug;90(8):870-881. doi: 10.1136/jnnp-2018-320106.

59. Gaetani L, Salvadori N, Lisetti V, Eusebi P, Mancini A, Gentili L, Borrelli A, Portaccio E, Sarchielli P, Blennow K, Zetterberg H, Parnetti L, Calabresi P, Di Filippo M. Cerebrospinal fluid neurofilament light chain tracks cognitive impairment in multiple sclerosis. J Neurol. 2019 Sep;266(9):2157-2163. doi:

10.1007/s00415-019-09398-7.

60. Jellinger KA. Neuropathological aspects of Alzheimer disease, Parkinson disease and frontotemporal dementia. Neurodegener Dis. 2008;5(3-4):118-21. doi: 10.1159/000113679.

61. Parnetti L, Farotti L, Eusebi P, Chiasserini D, De Carlo C, Giannandrea D, Salvadori N, Lisetti V,

Tambasco N, Rossi A, Majbour NK, El-Agnaf O, Calabresi P. Differential role of CSF alpha-synuclein species, tau, and Aβ42 in Parkinson's Disease. Front Aging Neurosci. 2014 Mar 31;6:53. doi: 10.3389/fnagi.2014.00053.

62. Petzold A. Intrathecal oligoclonal IgG synthesis in multiple sclerosis. J Neuroimmunol. 2013 Sep 15;262(1-2):1-10. doi: 10.1016/j.jneuroim.2013.06.014.

63. G.Defer, F.Daniel, chapter 14 (dementia). Book: multiple sclerosis: clinical and therapeutic. 2017.Elsevier Masson. B Brochet

64. Farina G, Magliozzi R, Pitteri M, Reynolds R, Rossi S, Gajofatto A, Benedetti MD, Facchiano F,

Monaco S, Calabrese M. Increased cortical lesion load and intrathecal inflammation is associated with oligoclonal bands in multiple sclerosis patients: a combined CSF and MRI study. J Neuroinflammation. 2017 Feb 21;14(1):40. doi: 10.1186/s12974-017-0812-y.

65. Bergendal G, Fredrikson S, Almkvist O. Selective decline in information processing in subgroups of multiple sclerosis: an 8-year longitudinal study. Eur Neurol. 2007;57(4):193-202. doi: 10.1159/000099158.

66. Genova HM, DeLuca J, Chiaravalloti N, Wylie G. The relationship between executive functioning, processing speed, and white matter integrity in multiple sclerosis. J Clin Exp Neuropsychol. 2013;35(6):631-41. doi: 10.1080/13803395.2013.806649. Epub 2013 Jun 18.

67. Sullivan, M. J., Edgley, K., & Dehoux, E. (1990). A survey of multiple sclerosis: I. Perceived cognitive problems and compensatory strategy use. Canadian Journal of Rehabilitation, 4(2), 99-105.

68. Callanan MM, Logsdail SJ, Ron MA, Warrington EK. Cognitive impairment in patients with clinically isolated lesions of the type seen in multiple sclerosis. A psychometric and MRI study. Brain. 1989 Apr;112 (Pt 2):361-74. doi:

10.1093/brain/112.2.361.

69. Grafman J, Rao S, Bernardin L, Leo GJ. Automatic memory processes in patients with multiple sclerosis. Arch Neurol. 1991 Oct;48(10):1072-5. doi: 10.1001/archneur.1991.00530220094025.

70. Archibald CJ, Fisk JD. Information processing efficiency in patients with multiple sclerosis. J Clin Exp Neuropsychol. 2000 Oct;22(5):686-701. doi: 10.1076/1380-3395(200010)22:5;1-9;FT686.

71. Einarsson U, Gottberg K, von Koch L, Fredrikson S, Ytterberg C, Jin YP, Andersson M, Holmqvist LW. Cognitive and motor function in people with multiple sclerosis in Stockholm County. Mult Scler. 2006 Jun;12(3):340-53. doi: 10.1191/135248506ms1259oa.

72. Parmenter BA, Shucard JL, Shucard DW. Information processing deficits in multiple sclerosis: a matter of complexity. J Int Neuropsychol Soc. 2007 May;13(3):417-23. doi: 10.1017/S13556177070580.

73. Benedict RH, Zivadinov R. Reliability and validity of neuropsychological screening and assessment strategies in MS. J Neurol. 2007 May;254 Suppl 2:II22-II25. doi: 10.1007/s00415-007-2007-4. Erratum in: J Neurol. 2008 Feb;255(2):309-10.

74. Barker-Collo SL. Quality of life in multiple sclerosis: does information-processing speed have an independent effect? Arch Clin Neuropsychol. 2006 Feb;21(2):167-74. doi: 10.1016/j.acn.2005.08.008.

75. Higginson CI, Arnett PA, Voss WD. The ecological validity of clinical tests of memory and attention in multiple sclerosis. Arch Clin Neuropsychol. 2000 Apr;15(3):185-204.

76. Benito-León J, Morales JM, Rivera-Navarro J, Mitchell A. A review about the impact of multiple sclerosis on health-related quality of life. Disabil Rehabil. 2003 Dec 2;25(23):1291-303. doi: 10.1080/0963828031001608591.

77. Zakzanis KK. Distinct neurocognitive profiles in multiple sclerosis subtypes. Arch Clin Neuropsychol. 2000 Feb;15(2):115-36.

78. Dujardin K, Sockeel P, Cabaret M, De Sèze J, Vermersch P. BCcogSEP: a French test battery evaluating cognitive functions in multiple sclerosis. Rev Neurol (Paris). 2004 Jan;160(1):51-62. French. doi: 10.1016/s0035-3787(04)70847-4.

79. Thornton AE, Raz N. Memory impairment in multiple sclerosis: a quantitative review. Neuropsychology. 1997 Jul;11(3):357-66. doi: 10.1037//0894-4105.11.3.357.

80. Achiron A, Barak Y. Cognitive impairment in probable multiple sclerosis. J Neurol Neurosurg Psychiatry 2003; 74 (4): 443-6.

81. Baddeley AD. Working Memory. Oxford University Press, Oxford, 1986.
82. Miller GA. The magical number seven, plus or minus two: some limits on our capacity for processing information. Psychol Rev 1956; 63: 81-97

83. Marié RM, Defer GL. Memory and executive functions in multiple sclerosis. Proposal of an adapted battery and preliminary results. Rev Neurol 2001; 157: 402-8.

84. Jennekens-Schinkel A, Van der Velde EA, SandersEA, Lanser JB. Memory and learning in outpatients with quiescent multiple sclerosis. J Neurol Sci 1990; 95: 311-25.

85. Thornton AE, Raz N. Memory impairment in multiple sclerosis: a quantitative review. Neuropsychology 1997; 11: 357-66.

86. Rectem D, Poitrenaud J, Coyette F, Kalafat M, Van der Linden M. Une épreuve de rappel libre à 15 items avec remémoration selective (RLS-15) In: Van der Linden M, and the GREMEM, eds. L'évaluation des troubles de la mémoire. Solal, Marseille, 2004.

87. Poitrenaud J, Deweer B, Kalafat M, Van der Linden M. Adaptation française du CVLT. Éditions ECPA, Paris, 2007.

88. Kenealy PM, Beaumont JG, Lintern TC, Murrell RC. Autobiographical memory in advanced multiple sclerosis: assessment of episodic and personal semantic memory across three time spans. J Int Neuropsychol Soc 2002; 8: 855-60.

89. Patti F, Amato MP, Tola M, Trojano M, Ferrazza P, Picconi O, et al for the COGIMUS Study Group. Cognitive impairment social functioning, and fatigue in patients with relapsing-remitting multiple sclerosis: the COGIMUS (COGnition Impairment in Multiple Sclerosis) study. Mult Scler 2008; 14 (Suppl. 1) : S265

90. Rao SM. White matter disease and dementia. Brain Cogn 1996; 31: 250-68.

91. Midgard R, Riise T, Nyland H. Impairment, disability and handicap in multiple sclerosis: across- sectional study in an incident cohort in More and

Romsdal County, Norway. J Neurol 1996 ; 243 : 337- 44.

92. Strober L, Englert J, Munschauer F, Weinstock-Guttman B, Rao S, Benedict RH. Sensitivity of conventional memory tests in multiple sclerosis: comparing the Rao Brief Repeatable Neuropsychological Battery and the Minimal Assessment of Cognitive Function in MS. Mult Scler. 2009 Sep;15(9):1077-84. doi: 10.1177/1352458509106615.

93. Corfield F, Langdon D. A Systematic Review and Meta-Analysis of the Brief Cognitive Assessment for Multiple Sclerosis (BICAMS). Neurol Ther. 2018 Dec;7(2):287-306. doi: 10.1007/s40120-018-0102-3.

94. Korakas N, Tsolaki M. Cognitive Impairment in Multiple Sclerosis: A Review of Neuropsychological Assessments. Cogn Behav Neurol. 2016 Jun;29(2):55-67. doi: 10.1097/WNN.0000000000000097.

95. Meca-Lallana V and al. Cognitive impairment in multiple sclerosis: diagnosis and monitoring. Neurol Sci. 2021 Dec;42(12):5183-5193. doi: 10.1007/s10072-021-05165-7.

96. Jougleux C, Joly H, Brissard H, Lenne B, François S, Hamelin F, Derache N, Morin J, Reuter F,

Colamarino R, Ruet A. French consensus procedure for neuropsychological assessment in multiple sclerosis. Rev Neurol (Paris). 2024 Jul 12:S0035-3787(24)00558-7. doi: 10.1016/j.neurol.2024.06.005.

97. Strober LB, Bruce JM, Arnett PA, Alschuler KN, DeLuca J, Chiaravalloti N, et al. A much needed metric: Defining reliable and statistically meaningful change of the oral version Symbol Digit Modalities Test (SDMT). Mult Scler Relat Disord 2022;57:103405. http://dx.doi.org/10.1016/j.msard.2021.103405.
98. Weinstock Z, Morrow S, Conway D, Fuchs T, Wojcik C, Unverdi M, et al. Interpreting change on the Symbol Digit Modalities Test in people with relapsing multiple sclerosis using the reliable change methodology. Mult Scler 2022;28:1101-11. http://dx.doi.org/10.1177/ 13524585211049397

99. Ruet A, Deloire MS, Charre'-Morin J, Hamel D, Brochet B. A new computerised cognitive test for the detection of information processing speed impairment in multiple sclerosis. Mult Scler J 2013;19:1665-72. http://dx.doi.org/ 10.1177/1352458513480251
100. Benedict RH, Amato MP, Boringa J, Brochet B, Foley F, Fredrikson S, et al. Brief International Cognitive Assessment for MS (BICAMS): international standards for validation. BMC Neurol 2012;12:55.

101. Maubeuge N, Deloire MSA, Brochet B, Ehrle'N, Charre'-Morin J, Saubusse A, et al. French validation of the Brief International Cognitive Assessment for Multiple Sclerosis. Rev Neurol (Paris) 2021;177:73-9. http://dx.doi.org/10.1016/j.neurol.2020.04.028.

102. Wechsler D. Wechsler Adult Intelligence Scale. 4th Ed. WAIS-IV San Antonio: Pearson; 2008.
103. War Department, Adjunct General's Office. Adjunct General's Office. Army Individual Test Battery Manual of directions and scoring. Washington, DC; 1944.

104. Godefroy O, GREFEX. Executive functions and neurological and psychiatric pathologies: evaluation in clinical practice. Solal: De Boeck; 2012

105. Naegele B, Mazza S. Le PASAT modifie': edition d'un test d'attention norme' chez l'adulte sain francophone. Solal; 2003.

106. Rousset J, Gatignol P. Inte're^t d'un nouvel e'talonnage de tests: re'flexion et mise en pratique autour de la batterie de de'nomination orale d'images DO80. Rev Neurol (Paris) 2014;170:A210. http://dx.doi.org/10.1016/j.neurol.2014.01.586

107. Havez J, Hermant P. E 'talonnage de la BETL (batterie d'évaluation des troubles lexicaux). Universte de Lille, France : Mémoire d'orthophonie ; 2009.

108. Benedict RH, Fishman I, McClellan MM, Bakshi R, Weinstock-Guttman B. Validity of the Beck Depression Inventory-Fast Screen in multiple sclerosis. Mult Scler J 2003;9:393-6. http://dx.doi.org/10.1191/1352458503ms902oa.
109. Alsaleh M, Lebreuilly R. Validation of the franc‚aise translation of a short Beck pressure questionnaire (BDI-FS-Fr). Ann Med Psychol Rev Psychiatr 2017;175:608 16. http://dx.doi.org/10.1016/j.amp.2016.06.015
110. Spitzer RL, Kroenke K, Williams JBW, Lo¨we B. A brief measure for assessing generalized anxiety disorder: the GAD-7. Arch Intern Med 2006;166:1092-7. http://dx.doi.org/ 10.1001/archinte.166.10.1092

111. Snaith RP, Zigmond AS. The Hospital Anxiety and Depression Scale Manual. Windsor: Nfer-Nelson; 1994.

112. Pardini M, Uccelli A, Grafman J, Yaldizli O ¨, Mancardi G, Roccatagliata L. Isolated cognitive relapses in multiple sclerosis. J Neurol Neurosurg Psychiatry 2014;85:1035-7 [jnnp-2013]

113. Sumowski JF, Leavitt VM. Cognitive reserve in multiple sclerosis. Mult

Scler J 2013;19:1122-7. http://dx.doi.org/ 10.1177/1352458513498834.

114. Leavitt VM, Tosto G, Riley CS. Cognitive phenotypes in multiple sclerosis. J Neurol. 2018 Mar;265(3):562-566. doi: 10.1007/s00415-018-8747-5.

115. De Meo E, Portaccio E, Giorgio A, Ruano L, Goretti B, Niccolai C, Patti F, Chisari CG, Gallo P, Grossi P, Ghezzi A, Roscio M, Mattioli F, Stampatori C, Simone M, Viterbo RG, Bonacchi R, Rocca MA, De Stefano N, Filippi M, Amato MP. Identifying the Distinct Cognitive Phenotypes in Multiple Sclerosis. JAMA Neurol. 2021 Apr 1;78(4):414-425. doi: 10.1001/jamaneurol.2020.4920.

116. Sperling RA,Guttmann CR,Hohol MJ,et al. Regional magnetic resonance imaging lesion burden and cognitive function in multiple sclerosis: a longitudinal study. Arch Neurol. 2001;58(1):115-121. doi:10.1001/archneur.58.1.11

117. Arnett PA,Higginson CI,Randolph JJ. Depression in multiple sclerosis: relationship to planning ability. J Int Neuropsychol Soc. 2001;7(6): 665-674.doi:10.1017/S1355617701766027

118. Patel VP,Feinstein A. Thelink between depression and performance on the Symbol Digit Modalities Test: mechanisms and clinical significance. Mult Scler. 2019;25(1):118-121. doi:10.1177/1352458518770086

119. Olek, M.J. Multiple Sclerosis. Ann. Intern. Med. 2021, 174, ITC81-ITC96.
120. Adolphs, R. The Neurobiology of Social Cognition. Curr. Opin. Neurobiol. 2001, 11, 231-239
121. Henry, J.D.; von Hippel, W.; Molenberghs, P.; Lee, T.; Sachdev, P.S. Clinical Assessment of Social Cognitive Function in Neurological Disorders. Nat. Rev. Neurol. 2016, 12, 28-39.

122. Marafioti G, Cardile D, Culicetto L, Quartarone A, Lo Buono V. The Impact of Social Cognition Deficits on Quality of Life in Multiple Sclerosis: A Scoping Review. Brain Sci. 2024 Jul 11;14(7):691. doi: 10.3390/brainsci14070691. PMID: 39061431; PMCID: PMC11274955.

123. Riazi, A.; Thompson, A.J.; Hobart, J.C. Self-Efficacy Predicts Self-Reported Health Status in Multiple Sclerosis. Mult. Scler. J. 2004, 10, 61-66

124. Grothe, M.; Opolka, M.; Berneiser, J.; Dressel, A. Testing Social Cognition in Multiple Sclerosis: Difference between Emotion Recognition and Theory of Mind and Its Influence on Quality of Life. Brain Behav. 2021, 11, e01925.

125. Kever, A.; Buyukturkoglu, K.; Riley, C.S.; De Jager, P.L.; Leavitt, V.M.

Social Support Is Linked to

Mental Health, Quality of Life, and Motor Function in Multiple Sclerosis. J. Neurol. 2021, 268, 1827- 1836.

126. Calabrese M, Poretto V, Favaretto A, Alessio S, Bernardi V, Romualdi C, Rinaldi F, Perini P, Gallo P. Cortical lesion load associates with progression of disability in multiple sclerosis. Brain. 2012 Oct;135(Pt 10):2952-61. doi: 10.1093/brain/aws246.

127. Roosendaal SD, Geurts JJ, Vrenken H, Hulst HE, Cover KS, Castelijns JA, Pouwels PJ, Barkhof F. Regional DTI differences in multiple sclerosis patients. Neuroimage. 2009 Feb 15;44(4):1397-403. doi: 10.1016/j.neuroimage.2008.10.026.

128. Dineen RA, Vilisaar J, Hlinka J, Bradshaw CM, Morgan PS, Constantinescu CS, Auer DP.Disconnection as a mechanism for cognitive dysfunction in multiple sclerosis. Brain. 2009 Jan;132(Pt 1):239-49. doi: 10.1093/brain/awn275.

129. Amato MP, Portaccio E, Goretti B, Zipoli V, Battaglini M, Bartolozzi ML, Stromillo ML, Guidi L,

Siracusa G, Sorbi S, Federico A, De Stefano N. Association of neocortical volume changes with cognitive deterioration in relapsing-remitting multiple sclerosis. Arch Neurol. 2007 Aug;64(8):1157-61. doi: 10.1001/archneur.64.8.1157.

130. Preziosa P, Rocca MA, Pagani E, Stromillo ML, Enzinger C, Gallo A, Hulst HE, Atzori M, Pareto D, Riccitelli GC, Copetti M, De Stefano N, Fazekas F, Bisecco A, Barkhof F, Yousry TA, Arévalo MJ,
Filippi M; MAGNIMS Study Group. Structural MRI correlates of cognitive impairment in patients with multiple sclerosis: A Multicenter Study. Hum Brain Mapp. 2016 Apr;37(4):1627-44. doi: 10.1002/hbm.23125.

131. Ruano L, Portaccio E, Goretti B, Niccolai C, Severo M, Patti F, Cilia S, Gallo P, Grossi P, Ghezzi A, Roscio M, Mattioli F, Stampatori C, Trojano M, Viterbo RG, Amato MP. Age and disability drive cognitive impairment in multiple sclerosis across disease subtypes. Mult Scler. 2017 Aug;23(9):1258-1267. doi: 10.1177/1352458516674367.

132. Johnen A, Landmeyer NC, Bürkner PC, Wiendl H, Meuth SG, Holling H. Distinct cognitive

impairments in different disease courses of multiple sclerosis-A systematic review and meta-analysis. Neurosci Biobehav Rev. 2017 Dec;83:568-578. doi: 10.1016/j.neubiorev.2017.09.005.

133. Brissart H, Morele E, Baumann C, Perf ML, Leininger M, Taillemite L, Dillier C, Pittion S, Spitz E, Debouverie M. Cognitive impairment among different clinical courses of multiple sclerosis. Neurol Res. 2013 Oct;35(8):867-72. doi: 10.1179/1743132813Y.0000000232.

134. Oset M, Stasiolek M, Matysiak M. Cognitive Dysfunction in the Early Stages of Multiple Sclerosis- How Much and How Important? Curr Neurol Neurosci Rep. 2020 May 22;20(7):22. doi: 10.1007/s11910-020-01045-3.

135. Mückschel M, Beste C, Ziemssen T. Immunomodulatory treatments and cognition in MS. Acta Neurol Scand. 2016 Sep;134 Suppl 200:55-9. doi: 10.1111/ane.12656.

136. Patti F, Morra VB, Amato MP, Trojano M, Bastianello S, Tola MR, Cottone S, Plant A, Picconi O; COGIMUS Study Group. Subcutaneous interferon β-1a may protect against cognitive impairment in patients with relapsing-remitting multiple sclerosis: 5-year follow-up of the COGIMUS study. PLoS One. 2013 Aug 30;8(8):e74111. doi: 10.1371/journal.pone.0074111.

137. Mattioli F, Stampatori C, Bellomi F, Scarpazza C, Capra R. Natalizumab Significantly Improves Cognitive Impairment over Three Years in MS: Pattern of Disability Progression and Preliminary MRI Findings. PLoS One. 2015 Jul 6;10(7):e0131803. doi: 10.1371/journal.pone.0131803.

138. Miller E, Morel A, Redlicka J, Miller I, Saluk J. Pharmacological and Non-pharmacological Therapies of Cognitive Impairment in Multiple Sclerosis. Curr Neuropharmacol. 2018;16(4):475-483. doi: 10.2174/1570159X15666171109132650.

139. Boeschoten RE, Braamse AMJ, Beekman ATF, Cuijpers P, van Oppen P, Dekker J, Uitdehaag BMJ. Prevalence of depression and anxiety in Multiple Sclerosis: A systematic review and meta-analysis. J Neurol Sci. 2017 Jan 15;372:331-341. doi: 10.1016/j.jns.2016.11.067.

140. Golan D, Doniger GM, Wissemann K, Zarif M, Bumstead B, Buhse M, Fafard L, Lavi I, Wilken J, Gudesblatt M. The impact of subjective cognitive fatigue and depression on cognitive function in patients with multiple sclerosis. Mult Scler. 2018 Feb;24(2):196-204. doi: 10.1177/1352458517695470.

141. Morrow SA, Rosehart H, Pantazopoulos K. Anxiety and Depressive Symptoms Are Associated With Worse Performance on Objective Cognitive Tests in MS. J Neuropsychiatry Clin Neurosci. 2016 Spring;28(2):118-23. doi: 10.1176/appi.neuropsych.15070167.

142. Tur C. Fatigue Management in Multiple Sclerosis. Curr Treat Options Neurol. 2016 Jun;18(6):26. doi: 10.1007/s11940-016-0411-8.

143. Berard JA, Smith AM, Walker LAS. A Longitudinal Evaluation of Cognitive Fatigue on a Task of Sustained Attention in Early Relapsing-Remitting Multiple Sclerosis. Int J MS Care. 2018 Mar- Apr;20(2):55-61. doi: 10.7224/1537-2073.2016-106. PMID: 29670491; PMCID: PMC5898916.

144. Pettersen JA. Does high dose vitamin D supplementation enhance cognition: A randomized trial in healthy adults. Exp Gerontol. 2017 Apr;90:90-97. doi: 10.1016/j.exger.2017.01.019.

145. Giovannoni G, Cook S, Rammohan K, Rieckmann P, S, Vermersch P, et al. Sustained disease-acti vity- free status in patients with relapsing-remitting multi ple sclerosis treated with cladribine tablets in the CLARITY study: a post-hoc and subgroup analysis. Lancet Neurol 2011; 10:329-37. doi:10.1016/S1474-4422(11)70023-0.

146. Rotstein DL Healy BC, Malik MT, Chitnis T, Weiner HL: Evaluation of no evidence of disease activity in a 7-year longitudinal multiple sclerosis cohort. JAMA Neurology 2015; 72:152-158. doi:10.1001/jamaneurol.2014.3537

147. Vaneckova M, Seidl Z, Krasensky J, Havrdova E, Hora kova D, Dolezal O, et al: Patients' stratification and correlation of brain magnetic resonance imaging para meters with disability progression in multiple sclerosis. Eur Neurol 2009; 61:278-84. doi:10.1159/000206852.

148. Benedict RH, Morrow S, Rodgers J, Hojnacki D, Bucello MA, Zivadinov R et al. Characterizing cognitive function during relapse in multiple sclerosis. Mult Scler. 2014; 20:1745-1752. doi:10.1177/1352458514533229

149. Morrow SA, Jurgensen S, Forrestal F, Munchauer FE, Benedict RH: Effects of acute relapses on neuropsycho logical status in multiple sclerosis patients. J Neurol 2011; 258:1603 1608. doi: 10.1007/s00415-011-5975-3

150. Bisecco A, Rocca MA, Pagani E, Mancini L, Enzinger C, Gallo A, et al. Connectivity-based parcellation of the thalamus in multiple sclerosis and its

implications for cognitive impairment: A multicenter study. Hum Brain Mapp 2015; 36: 2809 2825

151. Amato MP, Portaccio E, Stromillo ML, Goretti B, Zipoli V, Siracusa G et al. Cognitive assessment and quantitative magnetic resonance metrics can help to identify benign multiple sclerosis. Neurology 2008; 71:632 638. doi: 10.1212/01.wnl.0000324621.58447.00

152. Filippi M, Rocca MA, Benedict RH, DeLUca J, Geurts JJG, Rombouts SARB et al. The contribution of MRI in assessing cognitive impairment in multiple sclerosis. Neurology 2010; 75: 2121 2128. doi:10.1212/WNL.0b013e318200d768

153. Houtchens MK, Benedict RH, Killiany R, Sharma J, Jaisani Z, Singh B et al. Thalamic atrophy and cognition in multiple sclerosis. Neurology 2007; 18:1213-1223. doi: 10.1212/01.wnl.0000276992.17011.b5

154. Mike A, Glanz BI, Hildenbrand P, Meier D, Bolden K, Liguori M et al: Identification and clinical impact of multiple sclerosis cortical lesions as assessed by routine 3T MR imaging. AJNR Am J Neuroradiol 2011; 32:515 521. doi: 10.3174/ajnr.A2340

155. Mitchell AJ, Benito-León J, González JM, Rivera-Navarro J. Quality of life and its assessment in multiple sclerosis: integrating physical and psychological components of wellbeing. Lancet Neurol. 2005;4: 556-566.

156. Chiaravalloti N, DeLuca J. Cognitive impairment in multiple sclerosis. Lancet Neurol. 2008 ;7:1139- 1151

157. Turner A, Williams R, Bowen J, Kivlahan D, Haselkorn J. Suicidal ideation in multiple sclerosis. Arch Phys Med Rehabil. 2006 ;87: 1073-1078.

158. Boland P, Levack WM, Hudson S, Bell EM. Coping with multiple sclerosis as a couple: "peaks and troughs"-an interpretative phenomenological exploration. Disabil Rehabil. 2012 ;34:1367-1375

159. Bogosian A, Moss-Morris R, Yardley L, Dennison L. Experiences of partners of people in the early stages of multiple sclerosis. Mult Scler. 2009 ;15:876-884.

160. Halstead EJ, Stanley J, Fiore D, Mueser KT. Impact of Cognitive Impairment on Adults with Multiple Sclerosis and Their Family Caregivers. Int J MS Care. 2021 May-Jun;23(3):93-100. doi: 10.7224/1537- 2073.2019-091.

161. Amato MP, Krupp LB. Disease-modifying therapy aids cognition in multiple sclerosis. Nat Rev Neurol. 2020 Oct;16(10):525-526. doi: 10.1038/s41582-020-0383-x.

162. Sotirchos, E. S. et al. Effect of disease-modifying therapies on subcortical gray matter atrophy in multiple sclerosis. Mult. Scler. 26, 312-321 (2020)

163. DeLuca J, Chiaravalloti ND, Sandroff BM. Treatment and management of cognitive dysfunction in patients with multiple sclerosis. Nat Rev Neurol. 2020 Jun;16(6):319-332. doi: 10.1038/s41582-020- 0355-1.

164. Kalb R, Beier M, Benedict RH, Charvet L, Costello K, Feinstein A, Gingold J, Goverover Y, Halper J, Harris C, Kostich L, Krupp L, Lathi E, LaRocca N, Thrower B, DeLuca J. Recommendations for cognitive screening and management in multiple sclerosis care. Mult Scler. 2018 Nov;24(13):1665-1680. doi: 10.1177/1352458518803785.

165. Landmeyer, N. C. et al. Disease-modifying treatments and cognition in relapsing-remitting multiple sclerosis: a meta-analysis. Neurology 94, e2373-e2383 (2020).

166. Leavitt VM, Dworkin JD, Galioto R, Ratzan AS. Disparities in DMT treatment: Demographic and neurocognitive differences between MS patients currently treated versus not treated with disease- modifying therapies. Mult Scler Relat Disord. 2024 May;85:105508. doi: 10.1016/j.msard. 2024. 105508.

167. Manouchehrinia A, Larsson H, Karim ME, Lycke J, Olsson T, Kockum I. Comparative effectiveness of natalizumab on cognition in multiple sclerosis: A cohort study. Mult Scler. 2023 Apr;29(4-5):628-636. doi: 10.1177/13524585231153992.

168. Amato MP et al. Treatment of cognitive problems in multiple sclerosis. Cognitive functions and multiple sclerosis. MS in Focus. 2013.

169. Sastre-Garriga J, Alonso J, Renom M, Arévalo MJ, González I, Galán I, Montalban X, Rovira A. A functional magnetic resonance proof of concept pilot trial of cognitive rehabilitation in multiple sclerosis. Mult Scler. 2011 Apr;17(4):457-67. doi: 10.1177/1352458510389219.

170. Chiaravalloti ND, Moore NB, Nikelshpur OM, DeLuca J. An RCT to treat learning impairment in multiple sclerosis: The MEMREHAB trial. Neurology. 2013 Dec 10;81(24):2066-72. doi: 10.1212/01.wnl.0000437295.97946.a8.

171. ProCog-SEP: a cognitive remediation programme for people with multiple

sclerosis and reducing its impact on everyday life (French Edition); Paperback-May 13, 2020.

172. Sepulcre J, Vanotti S, Hernández R, Sandoval G, Cáceres F, Garcea O, Villoslada P. Cognitive impairment in patients with multiple sclerosis using the Brief Repeatable Battery-Neuropsychology test. Mult Scler. 2006 Apr;12(2):187-95. doi: 10.1191/1352458506ms1258oa.

173. Fisk JD, Ritvo PG, Ross L, Haase DA, Marrie TJ, Schlech WF. Measuring the functional impact of fatigue: initial validation of the fatigue impact scale. Clin Infect Dis. 1994 Jan;18 Suppl 1:S79-83. doi: 10.1093/clinids/18.supplement_1.s79.

174. Guelfi JD et al. Depression and depressive syndromes. Ardix Médical
175. Beck AT, Steer RA, Ball R, Ciervo CA, Kabat M. Use of the Beck Anxiety and Depression Inventories for Primary Care with Medical Outpatients. Assessment. 1997 Sep;4(3):211-9. doi: 10.1177/107319119700400301.

176. Wilson BA, Watson PC. A practical framework for understanding compensatory behaviour in people with organic memory impairment. Memory 1996;4(5):465-86. doi: 10.1080/741940776

177. Longley WA, Honan C. Cognitive impairment in multiple sclerosis: The role of the general practitioner in cognitive screening and care coordination. Aust J Gen Pract 2022;51(4):225-31

178. Benedict RHB, Amato MP, DeLuca J, Geurts JJG. Cognitive impairment in multiple sclerosis: Clinical management, MRI, and therapeutic avenues. Lancet Neurol 2020;19(10):860-71. doi: 10.1016/ S1474- 4422(20)30277-5.

179. Brochet B. Cognitive Rehabilitation in Multiple Sclerosis in the Period from 2013 and 2021: A Narrative Review. Brain Sci. 2021 Dec 30;12(1):55. doi: 10.3390/brainsci12010055.

180. Tacchino A, Podda J, Bergamaschi V, Pedullà L, Brichetto G. Cognitive rehabilitation in multiple sclerosis: Three digital ingredients to address current and future priorities. Front Hum Neurosci. 2023 Feb 23;17:1130231. doi: 10.3389/fnhum.2023.1130231.

181. Taylor LA, Mhizha-Murira JR, Law G, Evangelou N, das Nair R. Understanding who benefits most from cognitive rehabilitation for multiple sclerosis: A secondary data analysis. Mult Scler. 2023 Oct;29(11-12):1482-1492. doi: 10.1177/13524585231189470.

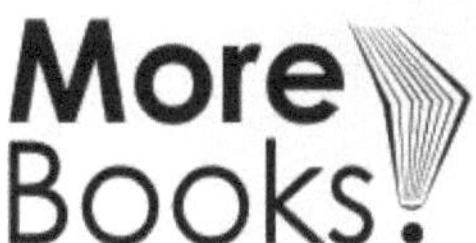

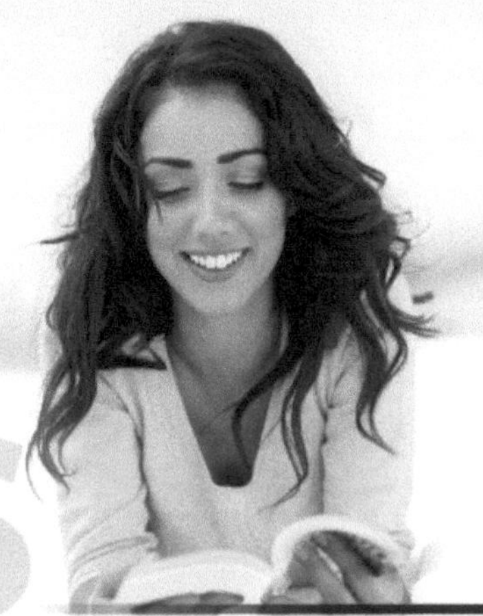

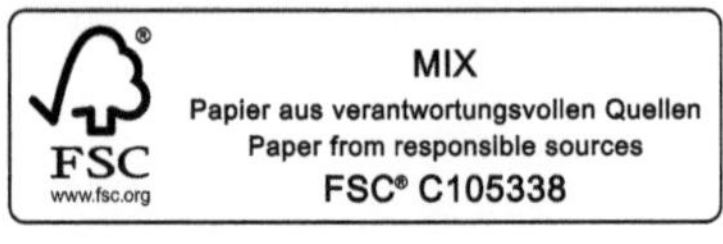

Printed by Books on Demand GmbH, Norderstedt / Germany